# Caring for People with
# Learning Disabilities

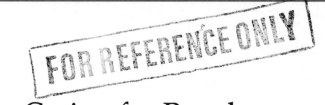

# Caring for People with Learning Disabilities

**Tom Tait MA, PhD, RNLD, RCNT, RNT, FRSH, MHSM, Cert Ed**
Senior Lecturer in Learning Disabilities,
Mary Seacole Research Centre, De Montfort
University, Leicester

**Nicky Genders MA (Learning Disability), BA(Hons), Dip Nursing, Cert Ed, RNMH**
Course Leader Diploma He (Nursing),
School of Nursing and Midwifery,
De Montfort University, Leicester

A member of the Hodder Headline Group
LONDON

This first edition published in 2002 by Arnold,
a member of the Hodder Headline Group,
338 Euston Road, London NW1 3BH

http://www.arnoldpublishers.com

Distributed in the USA by
Oxford University Press Inc.,
198 Madison Avenue, New York, NY10016
Oxford is a registered trademark of Oxford University Press

*British Library Cataloguing in Publication Data*
A catalogue record for this book is available from the British Library

*Library of Congress Cataloging-in-Publication Data*
A catalog record for this book is available from the Library of Congress

ISBN 0 340 80709 1

1 2 3 4 5 6 7 8 9 10

Commissioning Editor: Georgina Bentliff
Development Editor: Heather Smith
Production Editor: Jasmine Brown
Production Controller: Iain McWilliams
Cover Design: Terry Griffiths

Typeset in 10.5 pt Palatino by Phoenix Photosetting, Chatham, Kent
Printed and bound by Gutenberg Press, Malta

What do you think about this book? Or any other Arnold title?
Please send your comments to feedback.arnold@hodder.co.uk
http://www.arnoldpublishers.com

# Contents

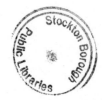

# Foreword

The word 'partnership' is now a very evident part of the everyday language of people who are involved in the process of providing care for vulnerable people. It is an expression that we have come to accept without a great deal of thought about the alternatives to partnership. The alternatives are characterized by closed thinking and a lack of shared vision and resources.

The alternatives to partnership may result in bad practice and a poorer service to vulnerable people but they are sometimes more attractive than partnership working because they are easier to operate. It takes skill; it takes knowledge; and it takes very positive attitudes to develop true partnership working, based upon values that recognize the integrity of people as individuals, regardless of the roles they play in the process of care. Whether they be users of services, family carers, practitioners or policy makers, the people involved in this endeavour have personal resources to offer which can only be improved by learning, by practice and by reflection.

That is what Tom Tait and Nicky Genders are inviting the reader to do in this book. They are authors with a broad history of success as teachers, practitioners and managers and they bring their wealth of experience to bear through the pages of this book. Typically, they have been able to relate the need for learning and the means by which to promote learning, to the delivery and practice of care. That is their gift, and that is what they have done successfully in this book.

In this book, Tom Tait and Nicky Genders have demonstrated an understanding of the complexities of disability. They do not underestimate the difficulties that confront people with learning disabilities, nor do they suggest that to care for someone with complex needs is a simple task. At the same time, they do not underestimate the problems that we all have in relating to the needs and personal perspectives of other people, especially where that person has learning or communication difficulties. By building upon the positive contributions that everyone involved in the process of care can make to overcoming or reducing these difficulties, however, Tom and Nicky have created a very positive framework for the practice, teaching and management of care.

I am therefore delighted to be able to commend this book to readers because it is uplifting and positive, like the authors themselves.

Colin Beacock, MA, RNLD, RGN, Cert. Ed
RCN Adviser in Learning Disabilities and Visiting Research Fellow,
Mary Seacole Research Centre, De Montfort University, Leicester

# Preface

This book aims to provide the new practitioner in the field of learning disability care with the knowledge to underpin their caring skills in a range of care settings. It will be of particular value for any practitioner who is undertaking a vocational study course or nursing foundation programme. The book is published against a backdrop of changing government policy towards people with learning disabilities with the publication of the White Paper 'Valuing People'.

The central theme throughout the book is the acknowledgement that a person with a learning disability is a person first and foremost and they will require a range of care interventions and levels of support to assist them with everyday living skills, no matter where they are living. Such interventions are driven by the need to work in partnerships with people with a learning disability themselves, their informal carers and professionals.

The authors have adopted a 'reader friendly' style, utilizing chapter aims and outcomes with suggested activities to help the reader reflect upon their developing understanding. The chapters are structured to introduce the reader to the philosophical base that can underpin care for people with learning disabilities and give practical guidance on how contemporary philosophies can be incorporated into everyday practice. Specific focus is placed upon the development of caring skills and their application in enhancing quality of life for people with learning disabilities.

Health gain and health promotion are key concepts that are addressed in some detail, together with cultural influences upon health status. Finally, the authors have chosen to highlight an informal carer's perspective on caring for a person with a learning disability, offering the reader valuable insight into the frustrations that informal caring can pose.

In summary, the authors hope practitioners working in either health or social care settings will find this book a valuable asset in helping them to develop appropriate skills, knowledge and attitudes to enhance their care practices. It is the acquisition of such skills that will help to ensure a person with a learning disability receives the appropriate individualized care that will result in positive and lasting gains to their quality of life.

Tom Tait
Nicky Genders
June 2002

# Definition of terms

Learning disability
: includes the presence of a significantly reduced ability to understand new or complex information and to learn new skills (impaired intelligence), with a reduced ability to cope independently (impaired social functioning), which started before adulthood, and with a lasting effect on development.

Informal carer
: carers who are usually family members of the person with a learning disability.

Paid carer
: a person who is in paid employment caring for a person/people with a learning disability.

People with learning disability who have complex needs
: people who, by virtue of their learning disability and additional physical, emotional or behavioural problems require a co-ordinated approach to meet their everyday needs.

# Acknowledgements

Mr Richard Jackson, OBE Hon Chairman, RESCARE (UK)
Mr David Matthews, author of the 'OK' Health Check. Preston:
Fairfield Publications.

# Principles of care for people who have a learning disability

## Introduction

This chapter aims to introduce you to a number of principles related to equality, diversity and anti-discriminatory practice to be considered when caring for people with learning disabilities and their families. Confidentiality will be explored as an important concept within care and will include the issue of abuse and protecting individuals from abuse. This chapter is designed to introduce you to the principles of providing good quality care to people with learning disabilities.

After reading this chapter you should be able to:

- appreciate the underpinning principles of individualized care to people with learning disabilities;
- identify ways to enhance the way you support people in your care;
- understand the importance of equality and anti-discriminatory practice.

You will be encouraged to explore the way you support people in your care. Activities are suggested that will help you understand why it is important to consider the following concepts when caring for people with learning disabilities:

- rights;
- privacy;
- dignity;
- independence;
- choice;
- fulfilment;
- diversity.

First, it is important to explore how, by adopting a philosophy of care that recognizes people with learning disabilities as people first, you can give high standards of care. You will also examine how, as a carer, you can offer an approach that is based on confidentiality, empathy and honesty.

The care you provide is underpinned by the belief that as a carer of a person with a learning disability you should:

- continually strive to protect the rights of the people in your care;
- always ensure you respect a person's privacy;
- maintain a person's dignity at all times;
- actively seek opportunities to promote independence;
- attempt, whenever possible, to help people lead more fulfilling lives;
- enable people in your care to make choices about their lives.

## Protecting rights

The United Nations (UN) declared a Bill of Rights in 1971 for all people with learning disabilities. As a member of the UN, the United Kingdom should be implementing the declaration. In practice, there are laws in this country, which are designed to run alongside the declaration. There are also social policies, economic constraints and prejudices that mean that part of the declaration may not be put into practice.

In 1996 the Disability Discrimination Act was introduced. The aim of this Act was to ensure that no person with a disability suffered any form of discrimination. This Act applies to people with a learning disability. Many organizations that provide services to people who have a learning disability have compiled a service charter that documents the rights of people who use their service.

This list contains various statements that relate to the rights of people with learning disabilities. They have the right to:

- be loved and accepted unconditionally;
- be educated;
- work;
- marry;
- have children;
- vote in a general election;
- live according to the laws of the country;
- choose where to live;
- choose with whom they wish to live;
- enjoy companionship;
- worship;
- express human emotion.

The question of rights is a complex area, but what must be remembered is that people with learning disabilities have the same rights as others in society but as a result of their disability may not be able to exercise these rights or may have these rights denied them.

## Activity

1. Make a note of any rights you feel are denied, for whatever reason, to people with learning disabilities in your care.
2. Think about the reasons why some of these rights might be denied and how you could help people to exercise those rights.

You may realize that it is not always easy to help people to exercise their rights particularly if these are in conflict with what the care environment is trying to do or if the right exposes the individual with a learning disability to risks and makes them vulnerable. Several factors may be restricting the individual from making choices.

- **Age**: children do not have the same legal rights as adults and therefore may not have the same opportunities to choose.

- **Severity of learning disability**: for some people with severe learning disabilities other people may need to make key decisions but you need to remember that people with severe learning disabilities can be helped to make choices in their everyday life.

- **Legal restrictions**: some people with learning disabilities, for example, those to whom certain sections of the Mental Health Act (1983) apply, may have their rights and choices restricted by law.

## Respecting privacy

When people live together, it is often difficult for privacy to be maintained. Assisting with personal hygiene and similar tasks may involve activities that you would normally do alone or not expect others to do for you. People in your care may need you to wash, dress and take them to the toilet but these activities should always be carried out with the individual's need for privacy in mind, in order to minimize embarrassment and discomfort. Specific examples of good practice in these areas will be discussed in later chapters.

A person with a learning disability will have a perception of himself or herself. The way we see and feel about ourselves is called our 'self-concept'. This is made up of all our beliefs and evaluations about ourselves. It is important to realize that having a disability may seriously affect a person's view of himself or herself.

As a paid carer, you have a duty to care for a person in a dignified manner that ensures their privacy is maintained. It is not only important to ensure people receive the appropriate care in privacy it is also important to treat the information we receive about them as private. This can be referred to as confidentiality. As a paid carer, you are duty bound to respect information and keep this information private.

The information you gain about someone in your care should enable you to make a judgement about what may be done for the benefit of the person. That knowledge should only be used for the purpose you required it for. It is 'privileged' knowledge and should not be given out. Disclosure of private information could seriously damage your relationship with the person in your care.

To summarize, people in your care should be treated with privacy. The information you gain about those in your care should remain confidential. If you are assisting a person with a learning disability to perform an intimate task, ensure you give them as much privacy as you would expect in a similar situation.

Remember your obligation to keep information private and

confidential. If a colleague asks for information about a person in your care, ask yourself, 'Do they need to know this information?' If this is the case, only disclose it if it is in the best interest of the person in your care. If you are unsure, do not disclose anything until you have spoken to someone who could advise you.

It is also important to remember that when a person dies it does not mean that you can then disclose confidential information about them. The information remains confidential.

The United Kingdom Central Council for Nurses, Midwives and Health Visitor's Code of Professional Conduct for Nurses, Midwives and Health Visitors (UKCC 1992) makes clear the nurse's role in relation to confidentiality.

Clause 10 reads, '. . . protect all confidential information concerning patients and clients obtained in the course of professional practice and make disclosures only with consent, where required by the order of a court or where you can justify disclosure in the wider public interest. . .'. This is good guidance for any health or social care professional working with people who have a learning disability.

## Maintaining dignity

The maintenance of dignity is closely related to the topic of the previous section. If you are to provide care that is dignified to people with learning disabilities, it is important to acknowledge that people are different. Just because two people with a learning disability may have the same condition does not mean that their care should be the same.

People are individuals in their own right. The care you provide will need to address the many different areas that, put together, make us who we are. These areas can be grouped as follows:

- psychological;
- physical;
- sociological;
- educational;
- spiritual.

To maintain the dignity of those for whom you care during your working day you should take the following points into consideration.

- Look for the human worth of the person with a learning disability. See the person, not the disability.

- Respect the racial and cultural origin of the people in your care at all times.
- Respect the gender and sexual orientation of the person in your care.
- Treating people with dignity will mean accepting their values and attitudes in a non-judgemental way.
- Regardless of circumstances, ensure that you respect a person's uniqueness and recognize their personal care needs.

In conclusion, by providing dignified care, you will be acknowledging that people are different and, as a carer, you must recognize these differences and deliver care that focuses upon personal needs. There are different dimensions to being human. Dignified care will therefore be based around the identification of personal needs in each of these dimensions.

## Independence

For many years, people with learning disabilities were cared for in large hospitals, often many miles away from the local shops and leisure facilities. The culture that existed was one of protection and containment.

People with learning disabilities were cared for under a regime that 'did' things for them; for example, people were bathed, fed, toileted, etc. Although people's physical needs were cared for, the regime did not fully recognize that people with learning disabilities could learn new skills that could help them become more independent and less dependent upon the care staff for assistance with daily living activities.

People with learning disabilities need to be taught skills that are relevant to enhancing their quality of life. Once these skills have been learned, opportunities should be provided that enable them to practice these skills.

## Enabling people to exercise choice

We will be faced with many choices during our working day. There are some decisions in life that are complex and require us to 'step back' and reflect upon possible courses of action. Even after a great deal of careful thought, we can still make the wrong choice. Hindsight lends objectivity however, what is important is the fact that it was our decision, and even though it failed, we can still learn from our mistakes!

Caring for people with learning disabilities is about meeting individual needs. We often place high priority on meeting needs but sometimes forget that exercising choice is also a need. Helping people to make choices and fulfil preferences is a key aspect in your caring role.

For many people with learning disabilities the range of choices they make in life may be limited. This could be the result of a range of factors including:

- **the care environment**: living with parents/carers who limit the choices a person can make or living in a group environment where choices are limited;
- **disability**: an individual with profound disability who finds it difficult to communicate their preferences verbally may have their choices limited;
- **attitudes**: carers may feel that an individual is not capable of making a choice or that they know what the person would choose anyway and therefore do not offer choices.

As a paid carer you will need to help people with learning disabilities to learn how to take more control of their own lives. This will require them to exercise choice. The very nature of your job emphasizes the requirement for you to look after people, to protect people from harm, and to care for them.

It is wrong for paid carers to allow people to choose a course of action and then deny them the outcomes of their choice. Not all choices will be easy to make and you may have to discuss the possibilities with the person in your care, as well as with someone whose involvement may help in decision making, for example, an independent advocate who can help a person make an informed choice.

In conclusion, caring for people with learning disabilities will require you to acknowledge that everyone, no matter how severe their learning disability, is helped to exercise some choice about their daily lives.

To enable this process to take place you will need to:

- assess a person's physical and mental capacities and levels of knowledge to enable you to have a clear understanding about how each individual can make choices;
- make available adequate information so that the individuals can make informed choices;

- promote opportunities that encourage people in your care to make choices within the context of acceptable risks and constraints of living with others;
- observe people's behaviour to guarantee that the care provided is balanced between people taking some control of their lives, the risks this involves and the possible impact upon others;
- safeguard any limitations to people with learning disabilities exercising choices;
- explain to the person why any choices have been limited;
- monitor such situations regularly.

## Protecting individuals from abuse

Many people who live within a care environment are at risk from abuse. Abuse can take many forms including:

- **physical abuse**: hitting, pushing, kicking, extremes of physical restraint and forms of physical contact that hurt the individual;
- **sexual abuse**: rape, indecent exposure and inappropriate touching;
- **emotional abuse**: including bullying, constant criticism, denial of rights, shouting and other forms of verbal abuse.

This is a short list and does not include all the forms that abuse may take.

As a paid carer, a key part of your role is to protect people in your care from abuse. Supporting people with learning disabilities to make choices and to communicate their wishes and views will help to minimize the risk of abuse. When people feel they can tell someone if they feel vulnerable or threatened, the risk of abuse can be minimized. Understanding the rights of individuals and valuing diversity can help the carer to understand how to prevent potentially abusive situations.

It is often assumed when we use the word 'abuse' that this means abuse of a person with a learning disability, by a carer. There is also a risk of abuse between care staff, as well as informal carer and their learning-disabled relative.

## Activities

1. Which of the following would you describe as abuse?
   - A service user uses racist comments to describe a carer.
   - A service user pushes another client who was annoying him.

- Members of staff send a service user to their room without their tea as a punishment.
- A male service user touches female staff in a sexually inappropriate way.
- Members of staff using degrading names for service users.

**All of the above situations are abusive.**

2. Discuss with work colleagues how you can help to identify and prevent potentially abusive situations within your care environment.

Care staff have a right to protection from abuse and people with learning disabilities have a right not to be abused by their peers. As a paid carer, you have a 'duty of care' to protect people with learning disabilities and your colleagues from abuse.

## Helping people to achieve greater fulfilment

We all have goals in life. Some people may have very few ambitions, others may have many and are determined to achieve all of them. We will further explore aspects of motivation later in Chapter 4. One theory that is commonly accepted as having great relevance when caring for people with learning disabilities, is Maslow's Hierarchy of Needs.

Maslow (1987) suggests that we have basic needs that need to be met before more complex needs can be satisfied. Look at the 'pyramid' illustration (Fig. 1.1). This is a representation of Maslow's hierarchy.

At the bottom are basic needs such as hunger and/or thirst. Once these needs are met, we are motivated towards higher, more complex needs. The needs at one level must be partially satisfied before those at the next level become important in determining our behaviour. Meeting basic needs is further discussed in Chapters 4 and 5.

Let us apply Maslow's theory to the lives of people with learning disabilities. Think back to the section on maintaining dignity. That section identified five areas that helped make us who we are. If you examine the hierarchy, you can see that these dimensions: physical, psychological, spiritual, sociological and educational needs are contained within its framework.

If a person's physical needs are not met, this will impact upon the other areas. As a paid carer, you will need to help ensure that the physical, safety, social, psychological and spiritual needs of those in

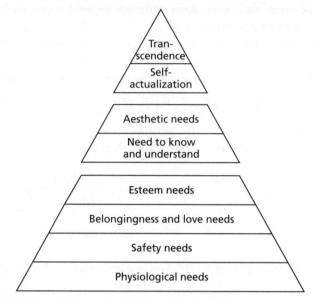

**Figure 1.1** Maslow's Hirerachy of Needs (Huitt 1998)

your care are met. Identifying needs and helping people to meet those needs will ultimately create the conditions where people can reach the top of the pyramid. These are peak experiences that are characterized by happiness and fulfilment.

## Activity

1. Using Maslow's hierarchy consider how your needs are met and who supports you to meet them. How can you can improve the way you support people with learning disabilities to achieve more fulfilling lives?

People with learning disabilities have the right to have such experiences too. Having a disability should not stop people having goals that will bring greater fulfilment to their lives. Goals are important concepts when planning care.

## Diversity

Health and social care professionals work in an increasingly complex, multicultural environment where there is a need for a deeper understanding of how our own culture influences the way we live. The cultural background and gender of a person with a learning disability will present a carer with many challenges.

It is suggested that people with learning disabilities seldom have their gender recognized. For a woman with learning disabilities this may prove a 'double disadvantage' as their individual gender needs will not be seen as important. Individual gender needs must be considered when planning and delivering care.

With regard to diversity and race, Tait and Higginson (2001) call upon the work of Blackman (2000), who argues that racial identity is not a stereotype, rather that it represents a significant aspect of social identity that can be usefully considered independently of other aspects of our personality.

Sir William Macpherson (1999) described institutional racism as something 'that can be seen or detected in processes, attitudes and behaviour which amount to discrimination through unwitting prejudice, ignorance, thoughtlessness and racist stereotyping which disadvantage minority ethnic people.' It is important to understand and accept that race is a complex concept and racial identity is not a stereotype.

Discussions surrounding race usually focus upon dark-skinned people. The racial identity of white people is rarely considered, yet white care staff will constantly make decisions that can profoundly affect the lives of people from ethnic communities in their care. Similarly, male carers may make decisions with good intent that can impact negatively upon the well-being of a woman with a learning disability.

The question of racial identity has significant implications for health and social care practitioners. The care you give a person with a learning disability must therefore be couched in an arena of equal opportunity and anti-racist care that acknowledges cultural differences. This will require you to understand and learn how to abandon conscious and unconscious racist attitudes.

Within the field of learning disability care, the current services available within the United Kingdom to people with learning disabilities from black and minority ethnic communities have developed through a process moulded by history and social policy. The history is fundamentally a white one and the social policies have evolved to meet the needs of white people generally. The constituents of good care principles for people with learning disabilities are grounded in a set of white, Western values. As services to people with learning disabilities developed, many services did not fully take into account the differing values and circumstances of people from the different cultures in today's society. Chapter 8 looks more closely at culture and how this may influence the lifestyle of a person with a learning disability.

## Conclusion

This chapter aims to introduce you to the concept of providing quality care to people with learning disabilities and the principles and values that should underpin that care.

A central theme is the promotion of understanding that the provision of quality care to people with learning disabilities is underpinned by a philosophy that requires you to recognize the human worth of a person with a learning disability, and adopt care practices that respect racial and cultural diversity.

People with learning disabilities may have many different, complex care needs. It is only by accepting their values and attitudes in a non-judgemental way that you will begin to develop skills further that help promote the person with learning disabilities as a valued, equal partner in their care.

## Additional activities

You may wish to complete these activities as evidence of your knowledge as appropriate to a number of care-related courses.
1. Summarize relevant legislation in relation to promotion of rights, equality and diversity.
2. Discuss the way in which clause 10 of the Code of Professional Conduct (UKCC 1992) impacts upon the role of the nurse.
3. Describe how people with a learning disability can be supported to make choices.

## References

Blackman, P.S. (2000) Exclusion by default. Combating Institutional Racism, Pride Park Derby. The Mary Seacole Research Centre. De Montfort University, Leicester.
Huitt, W. (1998) http://chiron.valdosta.edu/whuitt/col/regsys/maslow.html.

Maslow, A. (1987) *Motivation and Personality*, 3rd edn. New York: Harper & Row.

The Macpherson Report (1999) *The Stephen Lawrence Inquiry: Report of an Inquiry*, W. Macpherson. Cmd 4262. London: HMSO.

Tait, T. & Higginson, J. (2001) Partnerships and power in care. In: *Challenges in Clinical Practice*, Bishop, V. & Scott, I. (eds), pp. 117–135. Palgrave, London.

# What is learning disability?

## Introduction

This chapter looks at the concept of learning disability and how it arises. It explores one condition commonly associated with learning disability and identifies resulting health needs. After reading the chapter you will be able to:

- identify the major causes of learning disability;
- understand how learning disability can impact upon the family;
- appreciate how learning disability may affect an individual throughout their life;
- recognize one learning disability condition.

### Activity

Before reading this chapter spend a few moments writing down what learning disability means to you.

## History of learning disability

Learning disability is a condition that can result in pain and bewilderment for many families of which a member has a learning disability.

Moser (1995) traced the origins of learning disability and found that learning disability dates back to the beginning of human history. The concept of learning disability can be found in records as far back as the therapeutic papyri of Thebes, Egypt, around 1500 BC. Although somewhat unclear because of the difficulties in translation, these documents clearly refer to disabilities of the mind and body resulting from brain damage.

Learning disability is also a condition or syndrome characterized by a set of symptoms, traits, and/or characteristics. The terminology used to describe people with learning disabilities has changed through time. Historically, descriptions such as 'idiot', 'imbecile', 'feeble-minded' and 'moral defective' were used to classify groups of people with learning disability. It was not uncommon to have large hospital wards housing people with similar classifications. This type of care for people with a learning disability will be discussed later.

No matter what words are used to describe people with learning disabilities, having a learning disability does mean difficulties in learning and every day functioning. The nature of the learning disability will shape the levels and types of support the person will require to carry out everyday functions.

When working with people who have learning disabilities, it is important to remember that learning disability does not just affect the individual concerned. From identification, through treatment or education, parents struggle with questions about what caused their child's disability. They will want to know what the future holds. They may well be feeling guilty, experiencing a sense of loss, and be pessimistic about the future. Family members too will therefore need sensitive support and advice as they adjust to a life with a dependent family member.

## What causes learning disability?

Joseph (1997) identifies that learning disability can be caused by hereditary or environmental factors or a combination of both. During pregnancy, the developing fetus is vulnerable to a number of adverse factors that can cause brain abnormalities and result in learning disabilities.

Figure 2.1 shows the breakdown of the causes of severe learning disability that were identified by Susan Joseph. Generally speaking,

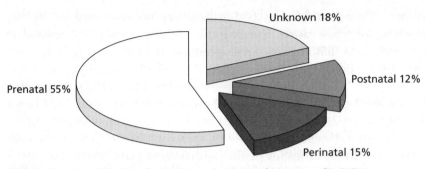

**Figure 2.1** Breakdown of aetiological causes of learning disabilities

prenatal causes are genetic factors, abnormalities or syndromes. Infections that happened during pregnancy will also fall into this category. Perinatal causes occur during delivery of the baby or shortly afterwards. A lack of oxygen, pressure on the surface of the brain and infections of the central nervous system come under this description. Postnatal causes are those that develop following birth and are not always apparent until the child displays some delayed development. Finally, there are causes that are classified as unknown as they do not appear to have a causative, genetic or biological factor.

## Genetic causes of learning disability

Through the study of genetics a number of specific disorders have been identified as being genetically caused. Genetic studies originated in the mid-19th Century when Gregor Mendel discovered, over a 10-year period of experimenting with pea plants, that certain traits are inherited. His discoveries provided the foundation for the science of genetics. Mendel's findings continue to spur the work and hopes of scientists to uncover the mystery behind how our genes work and what they can reveal to us about the possibility of having certain diseases and conditions. The scientific field of genetics can help families affected by genetic disorders to have a better understanding about heredity, what causes various genetic disorders to occur, and what possible preventive strategies can be used to decrease the incidence of genetic disorders.

Some genetic disorders are associated with learning disability, chronic health problems and developmental delay. Because of the complexity of the human body, there are no easy answers to the question of what causes learning disability, as this is attributable to any condition that impairs development of the brain before birth, during birth or in the childhood years.

The 'ARC', which is an American organization of and for people with learning disabilities and their families, refers to a study by Kozma and Stock (1992), who suggest that in 75% of children with mild learning disability the cause is unknown, therefore the field of genetics has important implications for people with learning disability.

As many as 350 inborn errors of metabolism have been identified, most of which lead to a learning disability (Scriver, 1995). The possibility of being born with a learning disability or of developing the condition in later years can be caused by multiple factors unrelated to our genetic make-up. It is caused not only by the genetic make-up of the individual, but also by the possible influences of environmental factors. Those factors can range from drug use to nutritional deficiencies to poverty and cultural deprivation.

## How often is learning disability inherited?

Because the brain is such a complex organ, there are a number of genes involved in its development. Consequently, there are a number of genetic causes of learning disability. Most identifiable causes of severe learning disability originate from genetic disorders. Up to 55% (Fig. 2.1) of severe learning disability can be attributed to genetic causes, making them the most common factors in cases of severe learning disability.

People with mild learning disability are more likely to have the condition as a result of environmental factors, such as poor diet, personal health habits, sociological factors such as poverty, access to health care and exposure to pollutants, rather than as a result of acquiring the condition genetically.

There is also a social dimension to learning disability. It has been suggested by Kurtz (1981) that status within society is attached to the role we play within that society. Having a learning disability can limit a person's everyday functions. This limited function will result in low status within the society in which the person lives. This low status, in turn, can reinforce a person's disability. Kurtz further suggests that learning disability can be perceived in two ways.

- The person with a learning disability can be regarded as a sick person.
- The person with a learning disability can be regarded as a developing person.

The first image is normally held by medical professionals and the second held by teachers, psychologists and, possibly, informal carers.

It is therefore important to understand that the sociological dimension to learning disability is centred on the role that people with a learning disability occupy within our society. The image that society holds about these people may be such that expectations are limited. The notion of learning disability in this sense is a construct of the society in which people with learning disability live.

Societies differ considerably throughout the world, therefore the social concept of learning disability too will be different. People with learning disabilities will therefore occupy different positions within different societies.

The following section explores one common condition associated with learning disability, Down's syndrome. Unfortunately, people who have certain conditions associated with learning disability often have general 'labels' attached to them; for example, people with Down's syndrome have been described as 'happy', 'always smiling', 'musical', 'good mimics'. It may be true that a person who has Down's syndrome may possess one or more of these qualities but such behaviours have nothing at all to do with Down's syndrome. People are individuals and they will develop their own individual personality.

While people with a learning disability who have a diagnosed condition may have similar health needs because of the common physical abnormalities associated with that condition, it is important to remember that such abnormalities will have a different impact upon each individual's life.

ARC (1993) produced a comprehensive guide to Down's syndrome and sections of the following description contain information drawn from it.

## What is Down's syndrome?

The estimated incidence of Down's syndrome is between 1 in 1000 to 1 in 1100 live births.

## How do children with Down's syndrome develop?

Children with Down's syndrome are usually smaller, and their physical and mental developments are slower than children who do not have Down's syndrome. The majority of children with Down's syndrome present with a moderate learning disability. Instead of walking by 12 to 14 months of age, as most other children do, children with Down's syndrome usually learn to walk between 15 and 36 months of age. Language development is also delayed.

## What do children with Down's syndrome look like?

Not every child with Down's syndrome has all the characteristic features; some may only have a few, and others may show most of the signs of Down's syndrome. Some of the physical features include flattening of the back of the head, slanting of the eyelids, small skin folds at the inner corner of the eyes, depressed nasal bridge, slightly smaller ears, small mouth, decreased muscle tone, loose ligaments, and small hands and feet. About 50% of all children have one line across the palm, and there is often a gap between the first and second toes. The physical features observed in children with Down's syndrome (and there are many more than described above) usually do not cause any disability in the child.

## What is the cause of Down's syndrome?

Although many theories have been developed, it is not known what actually causes Down's syndrome. Some professionals believe that hormonal abnormalities, X-rays, viral infections, immunological problems, or genetic predisposition may be the cause of the improper cell division resulting in Down's syndrome.

It has been thought for some time that the risk of having a child with Down's syndrome increases with advancing age of the mother, so that the older the mother, the greater the possibility that she may have a child with Down's syndrome. However, most babies with Down's syndrome (more than 85%) are born to mothers younger than 35 years. Current research is looking into the possibility that older fathers may also be at an increased risk of having a child with Down's syndrome. It is well known that the extra chromosome in trisomy 21 could either originate in the mother or the father. Most often, however, the extra chromosome comes from the mother.

## What health concerns are often observed in people with Down's syndrome?

Health issues will be addressed more specifically in Chapter 6, as all people with learning disabilities will have health needs. Certain conditions such as Down's syndrome will require a focus on specific aspects of health as a result of the physical conditions associated with the syndrome.

The child with Down's syndrome is in need of the same kind of care as any other child. The general practitioner, health visitor, district nurse and school nurse will provide general health care, such as immunizations, and offer support to the family. There are, however, situations when children with Down's syndrome may need special attention.

1. Between 60 and 80% of children with Down's syndrome have hearing deficits. Therefore, hearing assessments at an early age and follow-up hearing tests are indicated.
2. Some 40 to 45% of these children have congenital heart disease. This will have a bearing upon how much physical exercise they can undertake. Children play many physical games, but this condition may limit play activities and, consequently, how much a child with Down's syndrome will be able to play with non-learning-disabled children.
3. There is also a greater frequency of intestinal abnormalities in children with Down's syndrome; for example, a blockage of the food pipe (oesophagus), small bowel (duodenum), and at the anus is not uncommon in young children with Down's syndrome. These may need to be surgically corrected.
4. Children with Down's syndrome often have more eye problems than other children who do not have this chromosomal disorder; for example, 3% of children with Down's syndrome have cataracts which need to be removed surgically. Other eye problems including cross-eye (strabismus), near-sightedness and far-sightedness are frequently observed in children with Down's syndrome.
5. Another area of concern relates to nutritional aspects in some children with Down's syndrome, in particular those with severe heart

disease, who often fail to thrive in infancy. On the other hand, obesity is often noted during adolescence and early adulthood.

6. Thyroid dysfunctions are more common in children with Down's syndrome than in normal children. Between 15 and 20% of children with Down's syndrome have hypothyroidism. It is important to identify those individuals with thyroid disorders as hypothyroidism may compromise normal central nervous system functioning.

7. It has also been noted that there is a higher frequency of skeletal problems in children with Down's syndrome, including hip dislocation. Approximately 15% of people with Down's syndrome have neck instability. Most of these individuals, however, do not have any symptoms, and only 1–2% of them have a serious neck problem requiring surgical intervention.

8. Other important medical aspects of Down's syndrome, including immunological concerns, leukaemia, Alzheimer's disease, seizure disorders, sleep apnoea and skin disorders, may require the attention of specialists in their respective fields.

## Conclusion

This chapter has highlighted how learning disability is caused and the possible impact it can have upon the individual. You should note that having a family member who has a learning disability will also impact upon the lives of all family members in different ways. This chapter discussed the child with a learning disability but learning disability is an enduring condition that will impact upon a person in different ways as they become older. People's needs do not remain static and the following chapters will help you to plan care to meet these needs. Ways in which you can develop your caring skills will be explored to help you to enable people with a learning disability to lead healthier, more fulfilling lives.

## Activity

After reading this chapter, write down again what learning disability means to you? Has your definition changed in any way? Spend some time reflecting upon why you changed your mind. You may wish to ask colleagues what learning disability means to them. You will find that there are some common areas, but each person's experience of learning disability will be different and this, in turn, will influence their perception.

## References

Joseph, S. (1997) Causation of learning disability. In: *Dimensions of Learning Disability*, Gates, B. & Beacock, C. (eds). London: Baillière Turnbull.

Kozma, C. & Stock, J. (1992) What is learning disability? In: *Children with Learning Disability: A Parent's Guide*, Smith, R.S. (ed.). Maryland: Woodbine House.

Kurtz, R. (1981) The sociological approach to mental retardation. In: *Handicap in a Social World*, Brechin, A., Liddiard, P. and Swain, J. (eds), pp. 14–23. London: Hodder and Stoughton.

Moser, H.G. (1995) A role for gene therapy in learning disability. Learning disability and developmental disabilities research reviews. *Gene Therapy*, American Association of Mental Retardation **1**, 4–6.

Scriver, C.R. (1995) *The Metabolic and Molecular Bases of Inherited Disease*, 7th edn. New York: McGraw-Hill.

The ARC (1993) *Introduction to Learning Disability. Q&A*. Arlington, TX: The ARC.

# Communication

**3**

## Introduction

This chapter will explore the nature of communication both with people with learning disabilities and carers and some of the barriers to communication. By the end of the chapter you will have an understanding of:

- the components of verbal and non-verbal communication;
- barriers to effective communication;
- common disorders of communication affecting people with learning disabilities;
- alternative systems of communication for people with learning disabilities.

We begin to communicate from the moment we are born. As babies we communicate non-verbally through various cries and facial expressions and by the time we are five years old most of us have learnt to communicate our needs verbally.

For many people with learning disabilities communication is a difficult task. For some, the nature of their learning disabilities mean they will always find speech difficult and, for others, they may not have had the opportunities to develop effective communication skills. Later in this chapter, we will explore some of the issues around effective communication with people with learning disabilities.

## What is communication?

Communication is about sending and receiving messages. When two human beings come together, it is inevitable that they will communicate something to each other. Even if they do not speak, human beings communicate messages. Communication is so fundamental to human living that it occurs virtually all of the time in ways we do not even realise. Communication involves much more than talking, conversation or information giving.

As already mentioned, communication can be split into two main types.

- **verbal communication**: using the voice. A child learns from birth to respond to voices. This form of communication follows certain unwritten rules; such as if you ask a person a particular question, you expect some form of response.
- **non-verbal communication**: this is communication without the use of verbal language and is as important, if not more so, than the verbal part.

## Verbal communication

Verbal communication involves a whole range of activities. When you talk to someone your voice can indicate your culture, your mood, even the area where you were born or brought up. The way you speak can also reflect how you are feeling. You communicate all these aspects by adjusting various characteristics of your voice; for example:

- **pitch**: used to describe whether your voice is high or low; you might raise the pitch if you are very excited, when shouting or out of breath;
- **tone**: this refers to the quality of your voice; you might have a husky voice or make a harsh, clear sound. There are noticeable differences in voice tones between men and women;
- **pace**: this is concerned with the speed with which you talk; when excited you might talk very fast, but when bored or tired you may slow the pace of your speech;
- **volume**: how much noise you actually produce varies from whispering to shouting.

All of these characteristics combine to make your speaking voice, and therefore the words you say, more interesting. You are able to combine characteristics to produce the desired effect. Another person can pick up how you are feeling just from your voice and gain some idea of the type of response you want them to make.

Good communication is based on a message being sent, received and understood. Sometimes this is not as straightforward as it sounds; for example, if you were asked the question, 'Where do you live?', What would your response be? You would probably give an address or town. If you asked the same question and heard the reply, 'A pound of potatoes please', How would you feel? No doubt confused!

We usually know how to respond because we can understand the message. As a paid carer, it is important to recognize this because some of the people in your care may not fully understand what you are saying. People who speak different languages may also have great difficulty understanding everything that is said.

It is important that the person receives your message correctly and understands it. You can make sure of this by following certain rules for 'effective communication'. Ways of communicating effectively will be explored later in the chapter, but let us first look at non-verbal communication.

## Non-verbal communication

You can communicate non-verbally through drawing diagrams and painting, in music, or with your body. This is known as non-verbal communication. Some experts say that 90% of interaction between two people is communicated without words.

## Touch

A particular message is sent to the receiving person. This is another form of non-verbal communication that is very important in caring.

Touch is one of the oldest ways of communicating with others. As a carer, you may touch people as part of your daily routine and often on parts of their body that would not usually be touched, unless it was by someone very close to that person. In our society, there are unwritten rules about who you touch and where, and this will usually depend on the relationship you have with that person.

When talking about touch it is important to understand the idea of 'personal space'. This is the space around you which is your own. This space is usually an arm's length away from your body. If you stretch out your arm and make an imaginary circle around yourself, this is your personal space.

You only let the people you want into your personal space. If someone you dislike or do not know 'invades' your personal space, you may move, perhaps stepping backwards. You decide who to let into your space, depending on your relationship with them. Close friends and your family may be allowed to invade your personal space much more than strangers.

Touch involves 'invading' the personal space of another person and in a caring situation you may often touch people who are not close friends or family. You may wonder then why paid carers can usually touch someone they are caring for and 'break the rules'? As a paid carer, you are touching someone for 'health reasons' and you are allowed this contact because it is expected.

As a carer, you are in a privileged position in being allowed to touch someone in places where normally you would not be allowed. It is important to understand that some people in your care may feel a loss of privacy and dignity because of the amount of contact you may have with them. We look for consent when we touch someone. We often give eye contact and check we have their verbal or non-verbal approval. With people with learning disabilities, especially those with profound disabilities, this may be difficult, and as carers we must be very aware of this.

Personal touching is used when performing activities such as bathing; it is different to the kind of touch that communicates caring. Touch that reflects caring is very important to both the person being cared for and the carer. A touch on someone's hand or shoulder when they are distressed shows understanding, sympathy and compassion, and can ease a difficult situation. The carer who holds someone's hand or reassuringly pats them on the shoulder sends a non-verbal message of concern and caring. On most occasions, if you use this kind of touch to reassure a person you care for, it will be received gladly. However, some people see this kind of touch as an invasion of their personal space and would prefer you not to touch them at all in this way.

Touch also has different meanings in different cultures, so it would be useful to find out from other members of the care team, or the person concerned, what is acceptable.

## Clothes

The clothes people wear are also an important way of sending messages. The way you dress says something about you.

## Body position

The position of your body gives out particular messages too. This is included as part of your 'body language' because the body is also sending messages of its own, which may be quite different from what is being said verbally.

## Effective communication

People spend a great deal of time communicating because communication is the basis for building and maintaining relationships. It is important therefore that you learn the skills necessary for effective communication.

The skills of effective communication are of two kinds: the skills of sending messages and the skills of receiving. They take into account both verbal and non-verbal factors. When you are reading the following sections, keep in mind the information you have already been given regarding communication.

## Sending messages

Knowing what to say, when and where are all-important to communication. You cannot expect the other person to give you their full attention if you are trying to discuss something with them as they rush off to a meeting. Discussing a problem with your partner while he/she is in the middle of watching an interesting film is also not the ideal time.

You may also know exactly what you are trying to say, but for some reason, the other person is unable to understand. Accent and local slang may mean that you understand the message you are sending but the person receiving it may not. Speaking clearly will make sure your message is understood.

Making eye contact with the person you want to communicate with will allow you to check their response. You may need to look for signs of confusion, boredom or irritation, so that you can explain further. If you recognize any of these, you may need to stop and ask yourself, 'Is this the right time and place and am I making myself clear?'

Your non-verbal messages/body language have to match with what you are saying; for example, you would not give someone bad news with a smile on your face. This example is obvious but a more subtle example may be that your facial expression shows disinterest while you are trying to say something that you want others to be interested in.

You may also need to ask questions to check that the person has understood, such as 'do you know what I mean?'.

## Receiving messages

There are two parts to a message: the content and the feeling. When you are listening to someone, sometimes it is possible to hear but not truly listen. When you listen properly to a message you not only hear what the person is saying, but you also pick up the feeling behind the message.

In some forms of communication you only receive the content or the feeling in a message; for example, some people find it difficult to communicate on the telephone. This may be because it is difficult to pick up the feeling behind a message, but the content is clear. This is why, if you have a particularly emotional message to give someone, it is better to give it face to face. Sometimes when a person is very upset, it is clear how they are feeling but difficult to understand what they are saying.

It is also important not to let your own opinions and views get in the way. It is very easy to talk so much yourself that you stop listening to what the other person is saying.

To summarize, in this section we have looked at the nature of verbal and non-verbal communication and what helps you to communicate effectively. Understanding the components of communication will help you to understand some of the barriers to effective communication.

## Activity

Make a list of the barriers to effective communication you have experienced in your field of practice. These may include such difficulties as speech disorders or hearing loss. Identify some others that might affect a person's ability to communicate.

## Communication difficulties

We will now move on to look at some of the common communication difficulties people with learning disabilities may have.

Many people with learning disabilities have problems with their communication. The difficulties can include speech disorders, problems with non-verbal communication and social communication. Some of the difficulties may result from one or more of the following problems:

- cognitive impairment;
- undetected hearing loss;
- speech disorders;
- social learning.

### Cognitive impairment

Cognitive impairment is where the thought processes are affected so that there are difficulties with understanding and perception. Most people with learning disabilities have some degree of cognitive impairment and the degree may affect their ability to communicate effectively.

### Undetected hearing loss

Undetected hearing loss affects around 40% of individuals with a learning disability. If this is in a growing child, then the chances are that speech will be affected.

### Speech disorders

Disorders of speech can vary from mild disorders, where a stranger may have difficulty understanding the person, to a severe disorder, often affecting people with profound and complex disabilities. Disorders of speech can be caused by physical problems such as abnormalities of the face; cleft lip and palate are examples of this. There are also motor disorders which may affect the nerve supply and or the muscles that are needed for speech.

## Social learning

Social learning continues throughout life. In relation to communication we learn how and when to communicate from our families, peers, at school and at work. Each time we are in a new situation we learn how to communicate in that situation; for example, the first time we go to the cinema or theatre we learn to be quiet, to only talk in whispers and to listen to the film or play. If you had never had this experience or if no one had taught you about the 'rules' for communicating in this situation, you might behave inappropriately. Once we have learnt what is acceptable we then transfer this knowledge to other situations. We learn that we are also quiet in libraries and we can be much louder at a football match. For someone who has a learning disability, they may not have been exposed to the same social learning or they may not be able to transfer that learning to different situations.

Social learning is also a key to effective non-verbal communication. We learn body posture, social distance, personal space and a range of other non-verbal communication skills in this way. Someone with a profound disability may have difficulties in a number of these areas, which will affect their ability to communicate.

### Maximizing communication

Communication is a key through to a fulfilling life so it is important that, as a carer, you look for ways to maximize the ability of the person in your care to communicate. Communication difficulties among people with learning disabilities are not straightforward. A person who has a condition called Williams syndrome may have highly developed verbal skills but may be limited in their understanding or cognition. For individuals with delayed language development they may have difficulty with understanding and expressing words. Some people may also have difficulties with abstract concepts such as time or before and after. Individuals may use repetitive speech patterns called echolalia. This means they may repeat words or complex sentences but may not understand the meaning.

Understanding the communication abilities of the people in your care will mean you can begin to meet their needs. A full assessment of communication can be carried out by a professional speech and language therapist. This will give you an understanding of that individual's needs in relation to communication. The speech and language therapist may also suggest alternative systems of communication. These include some of the following techniques.

- **Sign systems**: the use of hand shapes, for example British Sign Language or the commonly used 'Makaton' Sign Language.
- **Symbol systems**: the use of symbols or pictures to represent objects, feelings or activities.
- **Objects of reference**: the use of everyday objects to represent something, usually an activity; for example a piece of towelling on the bathroom door, or a fork or spoon placed in the hand for mealtime.
- **Multi system**: a mixture of systems to meet the needs of the person in different settings and situations.

## Activities

1. Read the following care study and think about the ways in which you might help Sam to communicate more effectively. What type/s of communication systems do you think might be most appropriate for him and what do you think Sam's carers should consider in relation to communication?

   *'Sam Reed is 25 years old and lives in a small staffed unit with three other people. Soon after his birth it was noted that Sam had severe cerebral palsy, causing learning and physical disability. Sam uses a moulded wheelchair and needs daily physiotherapy. Sam has no speech but can understand most everyday words that are said to him. He likes staff to sit and talk to him and especially read to him. Because of Sam's physical difficulty he cannot turn pages of books and magazines over but he will look up at staff when he is ready for a page to be turned. He likes to point to pictures in the books but sometimes get frustrated if the care staff are in a hurry. The carers who work with Sam would like to help him to make more choices in his daily life. Sam often becomes upset and frustrated when he wants something and carers would like to encourage his communication so they know what he needs.'*

Discuss your thoughts with others in your work area or on your course. You may also like to find out more about the speech and language therapy services in your area.

2. Many people who have learning disabilities who are able to communicate verbally may have difficulty with their communication in a social setting. Take a look at the care study below.

*'Marie Staines is 35 years old and lives in a hostel with a number of other people. She moved there 10 years ago after living in a large hospital since childhood. She attends a day centre during the day and enjoys watching TV in the evenings. Carers who work with Marie both at the day centre and in the hostel often find it quite tiring when Marie is around. She has a very loud voice, talks constantly and often discusses quite personal issues loudly in public places. She also likes to hug staff quite tightly. Marie also joins in other conversations and 'takes over'. This leads to others around her becoming annoyed, so she has few friends as people think she is overbearing and bossy. Care staff often have to ask Marie to leave other people alone as she does not seem to notice she is annoying them.'*

Write down what you think the issues are for Marie's communication?

3. Make a note of strategies you might employ to support Marie to communicate more effectively.

## Conclusion

Communication is a complex issue affecting paid carers, informal carers and people with learning disabilities. Effective communication will enhance the lives and relationships of everyone concerned.

# Planning and delivering care to people with learning disabilities

**4**

Introduction

Developing caring skills

The care process

Person-centred planning

## Introduction

This chapter aims to introduce you to ways in which you can develop your caring skills. It will identify structures for the delivery of individual care to people with learning disabilities. Chapter 2 addressed the essential principles that should underpin the care of people with learning disabilities. This chapter focuses upon how you can deliver care based upon these fundamental principles.

When you have read this chapter you will be able to:

- explore ways you can further enhance your caring skills;
- understand how individual care is structured;
- assess and plan care using a systematic approach.

## Developing caring skills

You will have dreams and aspirations for your future and this will also be true for a person with a learning disability. The care assessment should therefore seek to ascertain not just the needs of the person with a learning disability in respect of the skills they lack but also what they feel may enhance their life.

Mayeroff (1971) described caring as a process that offers people (both carers and those in receipt of care) opportunities for personal growth. This means that you will, as well as the person you are caring for, learn new attitudes or feel new emotions and, possibly grow in confidence, as you plan together a course of action to achieve a jointly identified goal. The following section draws heavily upon the work of Morrison and Burnard (1991), who suggest there are certain major aspects to caring which are now discussed in relation to the care of people with a learning disability.

## Knowledge

Before you can care for a person with a learning disability you must know certain things. First, you must know that person. Just imagine a person whom you do not know very well asking you questions about your behaviour, how many times you go to the toilet in a day, can you read, do you have a sexual partner? You may feel these questions are very intrusive and you may be inclined to tell the person to mind their own business! Yet, relative strangers can ask people with a learning disability such questions and the details are recorded on a document that is available for all to see.

Think of your best friend. Your friendship developed because you got to know your friend and the more you learned about them the deeper your friendship grew. Perhaps you both shared an emotional event that resulted in you becoming closer. In relation to caring, you will have to get to know the person with a learning disability better, if you are to deliver care that is appropriate to them.

You will also need to have knowledge that you can use to the benefit of the person with a learning disability. You may find that sharing your knowledge with them will empower them to understand more about themselves. This process of enabling people in your care will facilitate greater involvement of the person with a learning disability in the care planning process.

When it comes to learning disability, the learning-disabled person is the expert. You may have an understanding of the causes and potential impact upon a person's life, but it is only the person with a learning disability who can empower you to achieve greater understanding of the affect their disability has upon them personally. This knowledge is unique and is personal to the person with a learning disability. Therefore, it is important to remember that you will have general knowledge about Down's syndrome but its impact upon a person's life will be exclusive to that individual.

## Patience

Morrison and Burnard (1991) further identify that caring for another person will involve taking time to develop the relationship. In your own life the relationships you have with others will not be constant. The relationship will fluctuate according to the intensity of the situation at that time. People can make us angry, happy, feel stressed or disappointed. Caring for a person with a learning disability can provoke similar feelings. In any care situation you will need to give the person with a learning disability time to 'allow' you to care for them. Just because you want to help a person with a learning disability to learn to feed themselves does not necessarily mean that they are happy for you to go ahead and do so. Your enthusiasm to care must be tempered with the need for the caring relationship to develop at a comfortable pace for the person with a learning disability.

You will need to exercise tolerance. Everybody is different and it is a requirement of caring that you must accept the person with a learning disability for who they are, not for what you may wish them to be. You can only hope the person with a learning disability will learn to like you. For this to happen requires tolerance, both with the person with a learning disability and you being patient with yourself.

## Honesty

Honesty involves being open or transparent. It will require you to tell the truth. To be honest with others requires you to start being honest with yourself. Lasting relationships are built upon honesty. Lies will damage any relationship. People with a learning disability require you to be honest with them. It is not always easy to be honest with someone, especially if the truth may cause him or her a degree of unhappiness or distress. This situation can also cause you to question whether you are doing the right thing. How can you care for someone when you are exposing him or her to pain by telling the truth?

In your life there may be a time when you will want to know the truth, no matter how painful it may be. By hearing the truth you will have been empowered to respond to the actual situation. Although people may tell you lies with the motive of protecting you from a situation, often the realization that you have been lied to is worse than the consequences of being told the truth.

To develop a therapeutic, close and lasting relationship with the people in your care will require you to evaluate your own thoughts, feelings, values and beliefs. Caring for people with a learning disability can challenge these, which can result in you not being open in your response.

## Humility

Morrison and Burnard (1991) state that to care for another person is a great honour. If a person with a learning disability entrusts you with their care, this involves you assuming responsibility for their care. This will place you in a powerful position and may result in you feeling good about yourself. In the case of a person with a learning disability, with a variety of complex needs, this responsibility may result in you having great control over that person's life. There is a hidden danger in this situation that such responsibility could mask your own inadequacies and lack of caring skills in certain areas.

## Hope and courage

Caring for people with learning disabilities is a challenging vocation. The very nature of caring suggests you believe in their ability to develop new skills and enjoy new life experiences. Caring is reliant upon hope. As your relationship with the person with a learning disability develops, you will know them more and become more aware of their hopes and fears. If you do not convey hope to the person with a learning disability, the chances are they will not seek you out for help or encouragement. Your caring relationship with them will ultimately suffer.

Caring for people with a learning disability is a unique experience compared to other branches of caring; for example, people are admitted to hospital unwell, receive care and are discharged in better health, often within a short space of time. Learning disability care requires a much greater understanding of people and an acknowledgement that, despite your best efforts, you may never achieve the care goals you aspired to, but only achieve a small step towards them. To care for people with a learning disability therefore requires considerable courage on your part.

It is also a brave act to share yourself with another person, as people can let you down. As you develop your caring relationships you will begin to share more of your life, your values and your beliefs with the people in receipt of your care. This mutual sharing can influence your life in a significant way and lead to more fulfilling experiences. But it is not without its disappointments. Caring for people with a learning disability does not mean just providing physical care but an inclusive process that is concerned with personal, familial, spiritual, environmental and emotional dimensions.

Unfortunately, the nature of a person's learning disability may mean they do not yet possess the appropriate life skills to reciprocate the relationship, and you may become frustrated that your constant efforts to develop a deeper, caring relationship are thwarted. This type of 'unequal' relationship demands courage from you. It requires the understanding that your self-disclosure may not necessarily generate self-disclosure from the person with a learning disability. In situations like this, you will require a reservoir of hope and courage as you develop the role of 'skilled fellow traveller' accompanying the person with a learning disability on their journey through life's many paths.

## The care process

To deliver care that is both individual and appropriate, it is important that you adopt a structured approach to care delivery. It is also important to have a documented plan of care that will provide:

- a baseline of information to help you to evaluate how the plan of care has impacted upon the quality of life of the person with a learning disability;
- a process to ensure the care you provide is based upon individual need;

- a system to make certain that information is readily available to other care staff when you are not at work;
- a framework for taking care decisions in partnership with the person with a learning disability, identifying care goals, providing care and measuring its impact.

Providing care to people with a learning disability cannot be carried out in isolation. Other care professionals such as speech therapists, occupational therapists, and physiotherapists too could be involved in delivering care. It is important that the activities of others are co-ordinated to provide an integrated approach to care delivery. The plan of care, therefore, can provide a framework for documenting the input of other professionals. As a professional carer you may well be the only person who is in daily contact with the person with a learning disability and your contribution to the care process is very important. You will be able to see, at first hand, how the input from other professionals contributes to the care process and inform them accordingly.

There are four main stages to the care process:

1. assessment of the needs of the person with a learning disability;
2. planning of care to meet the assessed need;
3. implementation of the care plan;
4. evaluating whether the care plan has met the care goal(s).

## Assessment

Previously under philosophies of care, the concept of the different dimensions of a person was explored. To make an accurate assessment of a person's life, it is important that the assessment you carry out takes these dimensions into account, in order to provide you with a balanced overall picture of the current need of the person with a learning disability. Care should not be assessed in isolation and the person with a learning disability must be viewed as an equal partner in the process.

## Activities

1. Using the following headings, identify two goals that you would like to achieve within the next 6 months.

|                     | Goal one | Goal two |
|---------------------|----------|----------|
| My physical health  |          |          |
| My happiness        |          |          |
| My family and friends |        |          |
| My general well-being |        |          |
| My education        |          |          |

2. Now ask a friend or relative to identify the same goals for you. The chances are that they might not identify the same goals that you did.

The case will be the same for a person with a learning disability. Often we will identify what we feel is important in our assessment. This will normally be based upon our knowledge of the person with a learning disability and what we think might enhance their life. It is equally important to ascertain what the individual's assessment of their own need is.

Other people can be involved in the assessment process, such as friends, relatives, teachers and day centre staff. They can make a valuable contribution to the overall picture of the current life of the person with a learning disability. This involvement can be invaluable when it comes to implementing the care plan, as everyone has helped to devise it. All people involved in the care of a person with a learning disability need to know and understand what is happening and who has responsibility for making it happen. A shared vision will result in a shared commitment to the care plan. Therefore the assessment process should involve all interested parties who can make a positive contribution to life of the person with a learning disability.

The assessment needs to be structured so that the information gathered is relevant to the needs of the person with a learning disability. Preprinted assessment forms are available. Some are designed to assess particular areas, such as a person's behaviour or a physical problem such as incontinence. These assessments can be very detailed and may require specialist knowledge by the person who is completing the assessment. A particularly helpful approach to delivering care is goal planning.

## Person-centred planning

## Strengths and needs

We all have particular strengths and needs in all aspects of our life; for example, you might be very good at cooking but not so skilled when it comes to ironing trousers! Just because you cannot iron very well should not stop you excelling in other parts of you life. For a person with a learning disability, they might have a disability that prevents them from walking very far but with the correct exercise, mobility aids and an adapted environment they could still achieve an enhanced quality of life through increased mobility.

It is important to remember that care plans too often only focus upon a person's deficiencies or problem behaviour. Just imagine how you would feel if people were constantly talking about your lack of ironing skills but appeared to take your excellent cooking skills for granted. You may feel devalued and to learn new skills or change your behaviour would help to motivate you. The assessment must therefore be a balance between what a person can do and what they have not yet learned to do.

Furthermore, once you start to make a list, you will find that a person with a learning disability will have many more strengths than weaknesses. Yet, the staff that care for them may only be aware of their weaknesses, as these are talked about most often. People with a learning disability often carry more 'labels', such as 'aggressive', 'dirty', 'anti-social', etc. A balanced assessment of strengths and needs can help to shift people's perceptions of the person with a learning disability from a negative to a more positive one.

## Planning goals

A goal is something we would like to achieve. Not all goals will be achievable at the same time. Some of our goals will have a greater impact upon our lives when we achieve them than others. The care plan must therefore have clear goals identified and a timescale for their implementation. Some goals will be more pressing than others. You will therefore need to agree with the person with a learning disability the key goals that are immediately achievable, which will form the focus of the care plan, and those which will need to be achieved over a longer period of time.

To achieve a goal in life may require us to take a staged approach towards its realization. For example, learning to drive a car requires us to build upon skills we have already learned, as well as learn new ones. The goal of passing our driving test will have been achieved by successfully undertaking a number of steps towards the final goal.

When planning care it is also important to make explicit, the criteria we will use to judge whether the step has been achieved; for example, if the person with a learning disability who you are working with, can cross the road using a pelican crossing in the manner they have been taught at 15 out of 18 attempts, is that an acceptable measure of success or is eight consecutive successful attempts a more accurate criteria? Such things will need to be considered as well as motivation.

We have already looked in Chapter 1 at Maslow's theory of motivation and you will need to take this into account when planning goals. The basic needs of the person with a learning disability will need to be considered at any planning stage. Furthermore, each step should be something that is achievable within a short time frame so that motivation can be maintained. Too often the steps are not small enough and the goal never appears as if it is being achieved. Small steps ensure the progress of the person with a learning disability can be monitored more accurately.

If you can plan small, achievable steps, the person with a learning disability will be able to build upon those successes with an increased motivation to achieve the care goal. The care staff too will be more motivated to work with the person with a learning disability as everyone likes to share in success. When we successfully realize our goals we are more inclined to want to achieve even more complex ones. Plan for success because success breeds success!

## Implementing the plan

It is important that everyone who will be working with the person with a learning disability knows what to do to achieve the goal. The following points are important in relation to how the plan is carried out.

1. **Write clearly**. The plan must be written in plain language, preferably in the first language of the person with a learning disability. Too often care plans contain professional jargon or abbreviations that increase the risk of it not being understood by everyone.
2. **Be explicit**. The plan should state clearly:
   • who will do what;
   • when it should be done;
   • where it should be implemented;
   • why it needs to be done.

This way all staff will know exactly what they are expected to do. It also serves as a written record that informs everyone, including the person with a learning disability, of their responsibilities.
3. **Keep to target dates**. Stipulate clearly when the plan will be evaluated. Identify who is responsible for organizing the review.

## Evaluating the care steps

This is the stage where a judgement is made based upon the criteria set out in the planning stage. If the step has not been achieved, then it may need to be broken down further. Alternatively, you may need to revisit the assessment and look for possible clues why the step was not achieved. Evaluation is an ongoing process. By listening and watching carefully for non-verbal cues you can build up an accurate picture of how the care plan is impacting upon the life of the person with a learning disability.

The care process should be a logical, systematic approach that is based upon key principles and values that help to guide the planning process. The collection of accurate knowledge about the person with a learning disability is only one part of the process. It is important for you to remember that the care process must not become a ritual. The central focus must be upon caring and the humanistic principles that underpin it.

Goal setting is a vehicle to help you structure your care in a way that makes it easier to harness the input of everyone and plan, together, achievable goals that can give greater life fulfilment to the person with a learning disability. Remember, the greatest service you will offer a person with a learning disability is care. The quality of care you provide is reliant not only upon you collecting personal, relevant information about that individual's life but also upon what you do with the information.

By actively involving the person with a learning disability in the care process you empower them to maintain as much control of their life as they feel comfortable with. You will begin to develop a wealth of knowledge and understanding of that person and begin to learn new skills as a direct response to their need.

## Conclusion

In conclusion, this chapter has introduced you to the concept of care planning and the need to develop a caring relationship with the person with a learning disability. The central theme identified is the need to work in partnership not only with the person with a learning disability but also with all the people who can make a positive contribution to their life. Goal setting can harness the enthusiasm and goodwill of others, and provide a systematic framework for delivering care that is person centred and aims to enhance a person's quality of life.

## References

Mayeroff, M. (1971) *On caring*. New York: Harper & Row.
Morrison, P. & Burnard, P. (1991) *Caring and Communicating Facilitator's Manual*. London: Palgrave.

# Skills for caring

## Introduction

Many people with learning disabilities need support with activities of everyday living such as eating and drinking, going to the toilet and keeping clean and healthy. In your role as carer, you will be in a position to give support to people with learning disabilities in your care to enable them to maintain their health.

This chapter will explore some of the skills required by you to assist the person with a learning disability to remain healthy. By the end of the chapter you will have an understanding of the skills required to:

- assist with eating and drinking, toileting and personal hygiene;
- carry out observations of vital signs and behaviour;
- assist in the administration of medicines and prepare an individual for practical procedures;
- understand the importance of health and safety while engaged in exercising these skills.

## Eating and drinking

Eating and drinking are a vital part of life. People need food and water to live but eating and drinking are also important social activities in our society. Many people with learning disabilities may need support with eating and drinking. Assisting people may also involve menu planning, food preparation and presentation and/or offering advice in one or more of these areas. It is important to have a basic understanding of nutrition to ensure that you can support individuals to eat a healthy, balanced diet. Advice can be sought from a dietician if you have any doubts about the dietary needs of those people in your care. In addition to understanding what foods are required for a healthy diet you may also be involved in feeding people within your care. There are a number of things you should be aware of when feeding people who cannot do this for themselves.

The presentation of food is just as important, even if the person does not appear to be aware of their surroundings. The person who needs feeding will be relying upon you for something which is quite personal. People eat at different speeds, some people like to chat during meals or perhaps take long pauses. For some people being fed may make them feel insecure and helpless. As a carer, feeding someone may be a regular activity within your daily routine. When you do something day after day, and during busy times, it may be easy to forget how the person you are feeding may be feeling. The following list comprises guidelines for feeding someone. Look through it and think about which, if any, you sometimes forget or skip when you are busy. You do not need to write down your thoughts but it is important if you are involved in feeding someone, that you offer an approach that is caring and empathetic, in order for them to get the most out of their mealtimes.

- Check food and drink are the correct temperature.
- Does the food look good enough to eat, and if not, can you expect the person to enjoy it?
- Is the person in a position that is not only comfortable for them but will also help with digestion and prevent choking?
- If necessary, is there a cloth or napkin to protect their clothing from spillages?
- Tell the person what the meal consists of.

- Offer food using the right utensils. It is not always necessary to feed someone a savoury dish with a spoon; a knife and fork may be just as suitable and may make the person feel better about being fed.
- Offer food slowly, allowing the person time to chew, swallow and, if they wish, chat between mouthfuls.
- Offer a drink between mouthfuls if the person wants it and between savoury and sweet courses, to prevent a mixture of tastes.
- After the meal make sure there is no food left around the person's mouth or on the clothing.
- After the meal offer the person the opportunity to clean their mouth or teeth.

Many people who are not totally dependent may be able to feed themselves using specially designed cutlery and crockery. There are numerous aids to eating and drinking such as spouted cups, broad-handled cutlery and non-slip mats. If you are working with people who need aids to enable them to eat and drink independently, it would be useful to find out where these aids are available and how to obtain them. If you have access to an occupational therapist, they would be able to give you this type of information, as will large branches of Boots the Chemist, and the British Red Cross Medical Aids Department.

## Assisting with toileting

Many people with learning disabilities may need assistance using the toilet. This can range from asking someone if they need to go, to giving full assistance to someone who uses incontinence aids. This section will explore some of the ways in which you may need to support someone with their elimination needs. Elimination is the term used to describe the removal of waste products from the body through bladder and bowel actions and through sweating and breathing. For this section, we are going to concentrate on the support someone might need with their bladder and bowel functions. When the body is functioning normally, waste products are removed in the form of urine and faeces. Urine is a straw-coloured watery fluid produced by the kidneys and contains some chemical waste products. Faeces or stools are soft but formed waste products produced by the bowel and may vary in colour and consistency.

Control of the bladder and bowel is generally learnt during child-hood. Most children have control over their bladder by around the age of 2–3 years, with bowel control a little earlier. Control means that the muscles have developed sufficiently and the messages from the brain can reach the bladder or bowel without problems. We consciously control our bladder and bowel and, during childhood, learn where the most appropriate place and the most appropriate time is to empty our bladder or bowel.

Many people with learning disabilities are incontinent of urine. This can be for many reasons. In order to be continent, there needs to be conscious control of the bladder. For many people with learning disabilities this is rendered impossible by their disability. It is impor-tant to recognize this, as it may be inappropriate to have someone on a toileting programme who will never be able to be continent. It may be more appropriate to manage this person's continence in an effective way by using aids. A specialist continence nurse can assess and advise on continence and ways to manage this.

Some people who have the ability to recognize when they want to use a toilet, may not have the physical ability to manage this. Many people with additional disabilities rely on carers to take them to the toilet. Occasional incontinence can occur when someone is wearing clothes they find difficult to manage. People who have visual impair-ment may also find 'getting to' the toilet difficult. Communicating the need to use the toilet may also be difficult for some people, and symbols or signs may need to be used. As a carer you need to be aware of the support you will need to give someone with their continence.

## Activity

Draw up a list of guidelines for assisting with maintaining continence for people with learning disabilities in your care.

## Assisting with personal hygiene and appearance

Many people with learning disabilities need help with meeting their personal hygiene and appearance needs. This can range from washing or bathing someone who cannot do anything for themselves, through to working with people who are able to maintain their own personal hygiene. Meeting an individual's personal hygiene needs can include washing, bathing or showering, cleaning teeth and mouth care, hair washing, shaving, dressing and grooming.

There are a number of considerations in this aspect of your role as a paid carer. You will need to understand the structure of the skin and the effects of different products on different types of skin. You will also need to feel confident with the actual skills, like bathing someone or shaving them. These may be skills that are new to you and you may need to learn these. You will need to take into account the needs of the individual, including their learning disability. A person who has Down's syndrome; may have dry skin and dry hair as a result of this syndrome; this will have implications for the types of skin care products used. Someone who is incontinent and has physical disabilities will probably require a different approach to someone who is physically active and continent. You will need to recognize cultural needs and these are covered in Chapter 8.

You will also need to take account of the individual's personal choice and of their gender. Being involved in this type of personal care requires an approach that recognizes the privacy and dignity of the individual.

## Activity

Imagine that you had to have full support to have your personal hygiene needs met. What would you want the carer to consider? Think about your own preferences and how you feel about your hygiene needs. How would you feel if someone left the bathroom door open when you were in the bath? Perhaps they might not help you to wash your hands after going to the toilet. If you are female, would you want a male involved with your personal hygiene, or if you are male, would you prefer a male or female to be involved in helping you with this type of personal care?

## Observation

Carers need skills in observation, particularly when working with people with learning disabilities. Many people who have a learning disability have difficulty communicating their needs and many find it difficult to describe their feelings. Skills of observation are therefore particularly important. You may need to make use of observation to record vital signs when someone is ill or to record changes in behaviour. As a carer, you will need to use a range of skills to observe patterns of behaviour or ill health in someone who may not be able to communicate effectively.

## Observing vital signs

Vital signs include temperature, pulse, respiration, blood pressure and, possibly, neurological assessment. Observing and recording someone's vital signs requires a range of skills and the use of equipment. You will need to be trained to undertake these observations but this section will help you to understand the need for such observations.

A number of factors can influence the body's ability to maintain normal functioning. These factors may include illness, physical activity or the environment. In the example of Emma, who has epilepsy, she becomes agitated before a major seizure; this is part of her epilepsy. During this period, her blood pressure rises and her rate of breathing may increase. Immediately after the seizure her body temperature may be raised as a result of the muscular activity during the seizure. This example highlights some of the physical changes that the body may undergo during a seizure. As a carer part of your role will be to recognize changes in normal functioning and report those to the appropriate person.

## Observing behaviour

Not only can we use observation to monitor changes in normal functioning but also to monitor changes in behaviour. When an individual has communication difficulties, subtle changes in behaviour can reflect how they are feeling. For those individuals who have regular episodes of challenging behaviour, it may be more difficult for carers to see beyond that behaviour and look for the changes that might reflect a change in health status. Observation requires the carer to be objective and not to make assumptions but to record what is seen or heard without assumptions being made.

## Preparing an individual for practical procedures

In order to maintain good health an individual with a learning disability may, at times, need to undergo practical procedures. These may include reading blood pressure, administration of an enema or suppository for constipation, drawing blood samples, administering an injection or changing a dressing. There are a whole range of practical procedures that a person with learning disabilities may need support with. Many people with learning disabilities have difficulty understanding the need for procedures and may feel frightened and unsure of what will happen to them. Part of the role of the carer is to support the person with a learning disability and help them to understand why they need to have the procedure, and what it entails. In giving this information, the key is to give it in a way that the person understands as much as possible about the procedure and the consequences. This may mean the use of signs or pictures for some people.

It is important as a carer that you understand the procedure and can answer any questions the person may have. You need to appear confident and not fearful yourself or this could make the person with a learning disability anxious.

It is not only support prior to the procedure that is important but also during and after. Explaining what is happening at the person's level of communication will help to reassure, and being available after to talk about any worries or answer any questions will support the individual. For some procedures there may be issues of consent. Generally, no one, by law, can give consent for another adult. The area of consent is not straightforward and can be very complex. You may need to discuss this issue further with colleagues in your workplace. There are guidelines on consent from people with learning disabilities.

## Consent

Consent is a complex issue. People with a learning disability have a right to autonomy and self-determination. They have the freedom to choose or refuse to participate in any care programme. In the situation of a person with severe learning disabilities, that person may not be fully able to exercise their right to self-determination because of the severity of their disability but you must acknowledge the person's autonomy and offer choices within their capabilities.

Severe learning disabilities does not automatically imply incapacity but decisions relating to consent may need to involve a range of people who understand the individual's situation and are able to act in his/her best interests. You will need to exercise caution if a decision made by a person with a learning disability is seen as wrong, as there is a danger the care staff may react in a paternalistic/materialistic manner. Paid carers must be aware of the subtle influences that relate to power, especially if they continue to use established methods for gaining consent.

Paid carers may be in a position of power and control and be seen as authority figures that can influence how the person with a learning disability comes to a decision.

## Assisting in the administration of medication

In many settings where people with learning disabilities live and work, carers are involved in assisting with the administration of medication. This can vary from assisting the qualified nurse, to undertaking the administration of medication following instructions from a doctor or pharmacist. It is important for anyone who assists with medication, to have an understanding of the principles of safe administration through an understanding of: legislative requirements; storage of medicine; side-effects; and routes of administration.

## Routes of administration

Medicines can be administered by a variety of routes:

- orally: by mouth in tablet, capsule or liquid form;
- topical administration: creams, ointments, patches and drops;
- inhalation: medication may be inhaled through the nose or mouth into the lungs;
- rectal or vaginal: suppositories and pessaries;
- injection: into muscle (intramuscularly) or under the skin (subcutaneously).

When administering medication or assisting, the following checklist of five 'rights' should be observed.

1. Right dose.
2. Right medication.
3. Right person.
4. Right time.
5. Right route.

Are you giving the right amount of the right medication to the right person at the right time using the right route? This checklist is important to have in your mind, whether you are the person assisting an individual in self-medication, whether you are giving medication prepared by someone else, or whether you are the person responsible for the administration of medication.

It is important that you are aware of any side-effects of medication an individual in your care may be taking. A side-effect is where an effect other than that intended occurs.

Many people with learning disabilities take medication over a long period of time and the unwanted side-effects from medication may have profound effects upon an individual's health status and on their behaviour. Particularly where the individual may have communication difficulties, you may need to observe for changes in health status and/or behaviour. When prescribing a medication, a doctor or pharmacist will be able to advise on possible side-effects. You can also find information about side-effects in the British National Formulary, of which there may be a copy in your care setting.

Storage of medication is also an important aspect. In the care environment there should be a safe, cool place to store medication. Medication should be checked to ensure the expiry date has not passed and labels should be easy to read.

If you are involved in the administration and/or storage of medication you should be aware of the following legislation:

- The Misuse of Drugs Act 1971;
- The Medicines Act 1968.

## Activity

Find out how medicines are stored within your care setting. Is there a policy available?

## Maintaining health and safety

While undertaking any caring skills, you must give consideration to health and safety issues. If you need to move someone, safe moving and handling techniques must be used; when helping someone to eat and drink, if you are involved in food handling, you must have undertaken food hygiene training; and when undertaking any clinical procedures, infection control procedures must be in place. Maintaining health and safety standards will not be something you do in isolation of other skills but will underpin all the skills you perform.

If you consider an example where you might use a range of skills to maintain health and safety standards in your workplace; this may be an occasion where you help to bathe, dress and give an individual who is immobile their breakfast. You will follow a range of health and safety procedures to ensure the safety of the individual as well as yourself. Some of those policies and procedures may include:

- safe moving and handling;
- infection control and disposal of linen and soiled items;
- the use of gloves/handwashing techniques;
- food handling procedures.

As a paid carer, you must be aware of the health and safety policies and procedures and work in accordance with these at all times.

## Activity

Take a look at the care study outlined below. What skills do you think you may need in order to care for this person effectively? What would be your considerations in delivering effective care?

*Jane is 23 years old and has multiple disabilities. She uses a wheelchair and needs support with all her daily living activities. She needs the help of two staff to move her from her wheelchair and she uses a hoist for bath times. She is on regular oral medication for epilepsy and suppositories for constipation. She is also incontinent and wears incontinence pads, which can sometimes make her sore. Jane tends to have seizures if she becomes constipated and needs diazepam administered, in some circumstances, if her seizures continue. Jane has help with eating and drinking and is slightly underweight. Jane communicates with those around her by nodding or shaking her head to direct questions. Jane is*

*able to make choices about the clothing she would like to wear and will*
*nod or shake her head to particular items of clothing if staff hold them*
*up for her to see.*

## Limitations to the carer's role

This chapter has focused on a range of caring skills, not specifically on teaching you these skills, as that usually occurs in the workplace, but on some of the understanding you will need to perform these skills effectively. Any skill you perform in the workplace must be within your limitations, you must have been taught or trained to carry it out, and you must feel confident that you can carry it out safely. Acknowledging limitations is an important part of all our roles and it should not be seen as a weakness but as a strength.

# Assessing health care needs

## Introduction

This chapter will help you to explore some of the issues related to assessing the health needs of individuals who have a learning disability. It is noted that people with learning disabilities have additional health needs that are not being recognized or met. A particular assessment tool, The OK Health Check (Matthews, 1996) will be used as an example within this chapter.

By the end of the chapter you should have an understanding of:

- the reasons why we need to assess the health needs of people with learning disabilities;
- the types of health needs people with learning disabilities may have;
- the OK Health Check assessment tool;
- the carer's role in assessment.

## Why do we need to assess health needs of individuals with a learning disability?

People with learning disabilities, like many people in the population, may have health problems additional to their disability. Down's syndrome, which was used as an example in Chapter 2, can be used to illustrate this.

It is the syndrome that has caused the learning disability but it may have also caused associated health problems. The person with Down's syndrome may experience poor circulation, dry skin, heart problems or a hearing impairment. They may also have a problem with the functioning of their thyroid gland and they could be prone to chest infections. Verbal communication too may well prove problematic, as the person may have problems explaining how they are feeling should they become unwell.

When people with learning disabilities live in the community they are registered with a general practitioner (GP) and follow the same procedures to gain access to their GP as anyone else. The GP makes up part of the primary health care team. This team includes a wide range of services and of course it is the GP who can refer a person on to more specialist services if necessary.

Other examples of where people with learning disabilities may need to use primary care services include screening services like breast or cervical screening. People may need to use the GP to monitor blood pressure, epilepsy or side-effects from any prescribed medication.

Many writers have noted for some time that people with learning disabilities have health needs that are not recognized. Howells (1986), Kerr, Fraser and Felce (1996), Turner and Moss (1996) and Lennox *et al.* (2001) noted in their studies that people with learning disabilities have health needs that include undiagnosed ear infections, cardiovascular problems, thyroid dysfunction, dental health problems, visual and hearing impairments and hypertension.

The report 'Once a Day' (NHS Executive, 1999) noted that up to one-third of people with learning disabilities have additional physical disabilities, often caused by cerebral palsy.

A physical disability like this can lead to:

- posture problems;
- difficulties with eating and drinking;
- constipation;
- incontinence.

It was also noted within this report that over 40% of people with learning disabilities have a problem with their hearing and many have eyesight problems. About one-third of people with learning disabilities may also have epilepsy and up to half may have additional mental health problems, including depression.

Despite these needs it has been found that many people with learning disabilities visit their GP less frequently than other members of the population. Therefore many of the problems go unnoticed. There are a number of reasons for this, including difficulties with communication which we explored earlier, poor formal support mechanisms and a lack of understanding of the health needs of people with a learning disability by members of the primary health care team.

One of the key difficulties in meeting health care needs is access to primary care services. A number of reports have recognized that people with learning disabilities may need extra help to access services in the community. The report 'The Health of the Nation: A strategy for people with learning disabilities' (Department of Health, 1995) stated that people with learning disabilities should have access to health promotion, health surveillance and maintenance and primary and secondary health care.

The report 'Once A Day' (NHS Executive, 1999), mentioned above, included recommendations for GPs and other primary health care team members to move towards meeting the health care needs of people with learning disabilities. In addition to these reports, the White Paper 'Valuing People' (Department of Health, 2001) recommended that there should be 'health facilitators' who can help to improve access to primary care services. Within your role as paid carer you may be required to help people to access services. This may include attending appointments with a person, giving information to primary care team members and helping the person to understand any treatment they may need.

'Valuing People' also made a key statement about the role of carers in meeting health needs, stating that workers providing support in '. . . social care settings have a responsibility for ensuring that an individual's health needs are met . . .'. This makes it clear that all carers have a responsibility to make sure that the health needs of those they care for are fulfilled, but how do carers identify what those needs are?

## Identifying health needs

It is important for the carer to have an understanding of the health problems a person in their care may have. These potential or actual problems could be linked to their learning disability, as in the example of Down's syndrome used earlier in the chapter, or they can be health problems that are unrelated. Unlike ourselves, many people with learning disabilities find it difficult to recognize the signs of ill health and may have problems describing these symptoms.

If someone has a problem over a long period of time, it might also be difficult to recognize when there are subtle changes in health status. As a carer, you will need to use skills of observation to note changes in health or behaviour. A change in behaviour could indicate a health problem. Behaviour may become challenging in people who have difficulty communicating their needs if they are in pain or discomfort. You may notice changes in sleep patterns or that someone has difficulty hearing what you have said. Knowing the people you care for and not making assumptions will help you to identify health needs. It is easy to put changes in behaviour down to someone's learning disability and not look for changes in health that may mean they are ill. Looking for these changes is often an informal way of assessing, but it is not always reliable. Another way to assess is to use a standard assessment tool.

The use of a standard assessment can help the carer to identify the health needs of people in their care with learning disabilities.

The OK Health Check developed by David Matthews (1996) is one such assessment tool. It is a comprehensive tool including the following components:

- body measurements;
- medication;
- experience of pain;
- circulation and breathing;
- urinary system;
- epilepsy;
- digestion and elimination;
- skin;
- physique and mobility;
- feet;
- oral hygiene;
- eyes and vision;

- ears and hearing;
- sexuality;
- sleep;
- mental health;
- lifestyle risks.

Each of the component areas has a number of questions to which the carer can answer 'yes', 'no' or 'don't know'. The 'don't know' response allows someone who may be more qualified, or another carer, to look at this component.

A handbook accompanies the checklist, which gives guidance on completion and suggests that the direct carer, key worker or other significant care team member should complete the assessment. This type of assessment checklist can help the carer identify health needs through a number of prompt type questions.

As a carer, you may not be able to make clinical judgements from the information you have gathered from such a checklist but you will be able to provide vital information about an individual's health status.

## Activity

Look at the care study below and identify what some of Martin's health needs may be. What type of support do you think you would need to offer to Martin in order for his health care needs to be met?

*Martin is a 68-year-old man who has severe learning disabilities and has physical problems that mean he uses a wheelchair. Martin lives in a small unit with five other residents who have similar disabilities. He is incontinent and relies on staff for all his needs to be met. Martin has impaired vision and no speech but communicates by nodding or shaking his head to simple questions. Martin has help with eating and drinking and is slightly underweight. Due to his lack of mobility and incontinence he sometimes has sore areas of skin. Martin can get quite distressed if the other residents are noisy and he likes to spend time alone in his room listening to music but this relies on staff wheeling him into his room. Martin takes regular medication for his epilepsy, which is well controlled, and for his constipation.*

Martin has recently started crying out and banging on the side of his wheelchair with his fist. The care staff have noticed he is eating less and less and is refusing drinks. His key worker feels he should visit the GP to see what the problem might be.

You may like to discuss this care study with a colleague or assessor/mentor.

## References

Department of Health (1995) *The Health of the Nation: A strategy for people with learning disabilities*. London: HMSO.

Department of Health (2001) *Valuing People: A strategy for people with learning disabilities in the 21st century*. London: HMSO.

Howells, G. (1986) Are the health care needs of mentally handicapped adults being met? *Journal of the Royal College of General Practitioners* **36**, 449–453.

Kerr, M., Fraser, W. & Felce, D. (1996) Primary health care needs for people with learning disabilities. *British Journal of Learning Disabilities* **24**, 2–8.

Lennox, N.G., Green, M., Diggins, J. & Ugoni, A. (2001) Audit and comprehensive primary health care assessment for people with learning disabilities. *Journal of Intellectual Disability Research* **45(3)**, 226–232.

Matthews, D. (1996) *The OK Health Check*. Preston: Fairfield Publications.

NHS Executive (1999) *Once a Day*, London: HMSO.

Turner, S. & Moss, S. (1996) The health needs of adults with learning disabilities and the Health of the Nation Strategy. *Journal of Intellectual Disability Research* **40(5)**, 438–450.

# Promoting healthy lifestyles

| Introduction |
| --- |
| Definition of health |
| Government guidelines on a healthy lifestyle |
| Difficulties for the person with a learning disability in maintaining a healthy lifestyle |

## Introduction

This chapter will explore the concept of health and the promotion of healthy lifestyles for people with learning disabilities. By the end of the chapter you should have an understanding of:

- what being healthy means to you;
- recent reports and legislation impacting on health;
- the ways in which carers can support healthy life styles for people with learning disabilities;
- some of the ethical considerations involved in promoting healthier lifestyles for people with learning disabilities.

Many people who think of disability often think of ill health. Being disabled does not necessarily equate to being unhealthy. People with learning disabilities should have the same opportunities to reach their own health potential as anyone else.

We need to begin by thinking about what being healthy means to us. What do you consider to be a healthy lifestyle? Is it being free from disease or illness, eating a healthy diet, never having to take a tablet, always being happy, and taking regular exercise, being the right weight for your height or not smoking or drinking excessively?

The responses to these questions will be individual, based on your health beliefs and your current state of health; for example, someone who has a problem which means he must take medication every day may not feel unhealthy, but if his condition becomes acute and he feels ill he might then describe himself as unhealthy. For people who have disabilities, they have often had their disability all their lives and do not feel that it makes them unhealthy but they may feel that a lack of exercise because of their disability does make them feel unhealthy. In order to understand what being healthy means, we need think about how we define health.

## Definition of health

A key definition of health that was published by the World Health Organization some time ago read: 'A state of complete physical, mental and social well-being and not merely the absence of disease and infirmity' (World Health Organization, 1947).

Although the definition takes on board the fact that health is not just about physical well-being but about mental and social well-being, it sees the concept of health as being a *complete* state of well-being. This is seen as an unachievable goal for many who have chronic ill health or disability. This recognition that health is more than 'not being physically ill' has continued to the present day.

## Activity

Write a definition of health that you think sums up what being healthy means to you. Do you think you could apply this definition to a person with a learning disability in your care?

Did your definition have different dimensions to it?

There is a widely held view that health has different dimensions to it. Some of the dimensions of health may include:

- physical health;
- mental health;
- emotional health;
- social health;
- spiritual health;
- societal health.

Health is therefore a concept that is personal and societal. We talk about our own health and what we feel makes us healthy but we also talk about health in society. The Government and other organizations publish targets for a healthier society and give advice on how, as individuals, we can meet these targets, which will, in turn, lead to a healthier society. The targets are also aimed at a societal level. Some things which impact on our health can seem out of our control. These include effects of pollution, chemicals and additives in foods, poor housing and intensive farming. It is acknowledged that not only individuals but also industry and governments have a responsibility for societal health.

## Government guidelines on a healthy lifestyle

A number of important documents have reflected the importance of maintaining healthier lifestyles: The 'Health of the Nation' document (Department of Health, 1992) set out a number of targets for the reduction of health problems in the following areas:

- coronary heart disease;
- stroke;
- cancer;
- mental illness;
- HIV, AIDS and sexual health;
- accidents.

These targets are examples of how health promotion can be viewed on an individual and societal level. If we take the example of coronary heart disease, we know that obesity, smoking tobacco and a lack of exercise can contribute to heart disease, so there is an individual responsibility to be aware of the risks and make lifestyle changes. The government also has a responsibility in relation to providing health-promotion materials, reducing tobacco advertising and offering NHS-based services for those who want to make lifestyle changes.

There are dilemmas though in relation to people making choices about lifestyle and the impact on health. What is your view on the NHS refusing heart bypass surgery to patients who smoke? Maintaining a healthy lifestyle is seen, therefore, as an individual, community and societal responsibility.

Soon after the publication of the 'Health of the Nation' report it was noted that, although it applied to the general population including people with learning disabilities, there were additional health needs amongst the population of people with learning disabilities and a further report made specific recommendations. 'Health of the Nation: A strategy for people with learning disabilities' (Department of Health, 1995) identified key areas for health improvements in the lives of people with learning disabilities. Chapter 6 highlighted some of the reports that focused on the health needs of people with learning disabilities.

When we think about the health promotion activities aimed at the general population, these may apply equally to people with learning disabilities, including healthy eating, reducing tobacco and alcohol consumption, taking regular exercise and avoiding high-risk sexual activity.

As a paid carer, you will have a specific role in assisting people in your care to maintain healthy lifestyles but this is not without its issues. People with learning disabilities may face a number of difficulties in maintaining a healthy lifestyle.

## Difficulties for the person with a learning disability in maintaining a healthy lifestyle

## Choice

People with learning disabilities may not be able to make choices about their health and their lifestyle. Many people with learning disabilities who rely upon carers have their meals provided for them. Relying on carers may also mean the opportunities for taking regular exercise are limited. This can also limit choices about other aspects of health too. In relation to sexual health, a person may understand what high-risk sexual behaviours are but not have the confidence to avoid these or may not have access to support. How do you think you or your colleagues would react if a person with learning disabilities in your care asked for a supply of condoms so that they could practise 'safe sex'?

Helping people to make choices, as in the example above, has ethical implications. Think about what you think some of these might be.

There are also ethical considerations when we are making choices for people. We are aware that being overweight can have a negative effect on health but we make a choice. We may know that our high-fat diet and lack of exercise is causing a 'weight problem' but we choose this lifestyle knowing the risks. For many people with learning disabilities this choice is taken away. If someone is overweight they may have their intake reduced and certain foods limited without any consultation.

In order to make choices we need information, and people with learning disabilities need to be able to access appropriate information.

## Access to information

Much of the health promotion material we see comes in written or visual form. There are television advertisements for giving up smoking; you can pick up leaflets about healthy eating at your doctor's surgery or read about health and fitness in magazines and newspapers. If we want to read about healthy lifestyles, we are surrounded by health promotion literature. Many people with learning disabilities have difficulty with reading and may not understand the way in which some of this information is provided. There are specific resources aimed at helping people with learning disabilities and we have listed some of these at the end of the chapter.

It is not only information in a written form that people may find difficulty with but also information that is given verbally. A doctor, nurse or carer may feel they have explained a health issue clearly but the person with a learning disability may have some difficulties understanding some of the concepts. As a carer, you need to be sure that information is clear and in a form that person can understand. This may mean you assisting health care professionals to communicate effectively with the person in your care.

## Activity

Next time you are in your local health centre pick up some health education leaflets. They could be on healthy eating, sexual health or smoking. Look at the leaflet as if you are the person you care for, who has learning disabilities. Consider whether you think the leaflet is easy to understand and how it could be made more accessible for people with learning disabilities.

## Finance

Having a healthy lifestyle is not always easy on a limited budget. Many people with learning disabilities live on a very limited budget and as a carer, you will need to explore cost-effective ways to maintain a healthy lifestyle; for example, for some people taking regular exercise means going to the gym a couple of times a week but this could be impossible on a limited budget. Walking is free and an excellent form of exercise for many. Do you have the staff available to encourage this type of activity?

## Activity

Think about the ways in which you could promote healthy lifestyles without any additional funds.

There are, as you will have seen, a number of challenges implicit in promoting healthy lifestyles for people with learning disabilities. You may be involved in supporting people to make a number of choices about their lifestyle and these are not always straightforward.

## Activity

Look at the care study below. What do you think Mary's needs might be in relation to health promotion? How, as a carer, do you think you could support Mary to make healthy choices?

*Mary Smith is a 35-year-old woman who has Down's syndrome. She has a part time job in a café and lives with three other people in a house supported by care workers who visit each day. Mary's leisure time consists mainly of watching TV or looking at magazines. Mary has a relationship with a man who lives close by and they have talked to support workers about getting married. They enjoy going for walks together but cannot go too far as Mary gets quite breathless. Mary enjoys preparing simple meals for her and the other residents of the house and she takes a packed lunch with her to work. Mary has a problem with her weight. She has been overweight for a number of years and her GP is becoming increasingly concerned about her health. Mary often has chest infections in the winter months and her circulation is poor. She takes no regular medication other than the contraceptive pill but is often prescribed antibiotic medication during the winter. Although Mary will talk to female support workers about her health, she is wary of male workers and prefers not to talk to them about 'personal' matters.*

There are a number of considerations here and you may find it useful to discuss your thoughts with a colleague, mentor or assessor.

## Conclusion

Health promotion is a key role for any paid carer. It is important to acknowledge some of the difficulties and work necessary to support people with learning disabilities to have healthy lifestyles, but also to recognize that people do make choices and that choice needs to be 'informed'. That is, that people with learning disabilities should have all the information in a way they can understand and they want to make a choice.

## References

Department of Health (1992) *The Health of the Nation*. London: HMSO.

Department of Health (1995) *The Health of the Nation: A strategy for people with learning disabilities*. London: HMSO.

World Health Organization (1947) *Constitution*, Geneva: World Health Organization.

## Publications suitable for people with learning disabilities

Band R. (1997) *Getting Better—How people with learning disabilities can get the best from their GP*. Brighton: Pavilion Publishing. Consists of a video, booklet and handouts. Available from: Pavilion Publishing Ltd., FREEPOST (BR458) 8 St George's Place, Brighton, East Sussex BN1 4ZZ.

Band R. (1998) *Food, Keep clean, Safety in the Home, Epilepsy* and *Coming for a Drink?* The Healthy Living Series. London: Elfrida Society. Five booklets available from: The Elfrida Society, The Tom Blythe Centre, 34 Islington Park Street, London N1 1PX.

BILD Publications (1997) *If you are Ill, Looking after your Teeth, Coping with Stress, Eating and Drinking, Breathe Easy, Alcohol and Smoking, Exercise, Seeing and Hearing, Sex, Using Medicine Safely*. Your Good Health Series. Plymouth: BILD publications. Ten booklets available from: BILD Publications, Plymbridge Distributors, Plymbridge House, Estover Road, Plymouth PL6 7PZ.

Department of Health (1998) *The Healthy Way*. London: HMSO. An illustrated easy-to-read booklet, a cassette and a poster suitable for service users and those who support them. Available from: Department of Health, PO Box 410, Wetherby, Yorkshire LS23 7LN.

Dodd K. & Brunker J. (1998) *Feeling Poorly*. Brighton: Pavilion Publishing. A large pocketed ring binder providing a training programme and resources for people with learning disabilities and their support workers. Available from: Pavilion Publishing Ltd., FREEPOST (BR458) 8 St George's Place, Brighton, East Sussex BN1 4ZZ.

Health Education Authority (1995) *Health Related Resources for People with Learning Disabilities*. London: HMSO. Available from: Health Education Authority, Hamilton House, Mabledon Place, London WC1H 9TX.

Hollins S., Bernal J. & Gregory M. (1996) *Going to the Doctor*. Books Beyond Words Series. London: Royal College of Psychiatrists. Available from: Royal College of Psychiatrists, 17 Belgrave Square, London SW1X 8PG.

Hollins S., Avis A. & Cheverton, S. (1998) *Going into Hospital*. Books Beyond Words Series. London: Royal College of Psychiatrists. Available from: Royal College of Psychiatrists, 17 Belgrave Square, London SW1X 8PG.

Hollins S., Bernal J. & Gregory M. (1998) *Going to Outpatients*. Books Beyond Words Series. London: Royal College of Psychiatrists. Available from: Royal College of Psychiatrists, 17 Belgrave Square, London SW1X 8PG.

Paul A. *Epilepsy and You*. Brighton: Pavilion Publishing. Video assisted training package. Available from: Pavilion Publishing Ltd., FREEPOST (BR458) 8 St George's Place, Brighton, East Sussex BN1 4ZZ.

Speak up Self Advocacy (1998) *How to go into Hospital*. Brighton: Pavilion Publishing. Video. Available from: Pavilion Publishing Ltd., FREEPOST (BR458) 8 St George's Place, Brighton, East Sussex BN1 4ZZ.

# Delivering culturally appropriate care to people with learning disabilities

**8**

## Introduction

This chapter is designed to heighten your awareness of the importance of delivering care that is sensitive to individual cultural needs. One chapter alone cannot cover every single aspect of each religious or cultural group's customs that may impact upon a person's life, but this chapter aims to give you valuable insight into the rich diversity of customs and practices of the main ethnic minority groups within our society.

At the end of the chapter you will be able to:

• understand the importance culture plays in a person's life;
• appreciate the 'double disadvantage' a person with a learning disability can have when they belong to a minority ethnic community;
• identify components of institutional racism.

## Activity

Please complete this small test before reading the chapter.

1. How would you help a Hindu woman to dress or undress?
2. Which cultural group celebrates Chanukah and Yom Kippur?
3. What arrangements for washing are necessary for Sikhs?
4. What do Muslims generally believe about contraception?
5. Whom would you contact to give comfort to a Sikh who is dying?
6. By which of a Muslim's names would you address him or her?
7. Which cultural group celebrates Wesak?
8. Which cultural group considers the cow as a sacred animal?
9. Eating pork is strictly forbidden in which cultural group?
10. Which cultural group has a raised incidence of high blood pressure compared to other groups in society?

## Setting the scene

Although it is recognized that ethnicity is an important issue for people who plan health or social care services, its reference to people with learning disabilities is fairly recent. McMillan (1992) suggested that there are many misconceptions regarding ethnicity and people with learning disabilities. Many generalizations are made about attitudes of particular groups, and this is true of people from ethnic minority communities; for example, stereotypical attitudes of Asian people being a homogeneous group, who live in large extended families caring 'for their own' and dominated by men are commonplace.

Baxter *et al.* (1990) argued that we live in a multiracial society yet most of the key literature on developing services for people with learning disabilities has ignored this fact. The particular experiences, circumstances and needs of Asian children and adults with learning disabilities and their families are ignored or assumed to be the same as those of their white counterparts.

Ayer (1997) suggested that many Asian families with a learning-disabled family member had limited knowledge of the support services available. It has also been found that mothers of children who have a learning disability from minority ethnic communities can be isolated and lacking in support compared to white mothers. Historically, people with a learning disability from a minority ethnic community generally have not made the same use of services compared to their white counterparts. Sadly, they have often been blamed for this behaviour.

Yet it is not surprising that people failed to make use of services that only catered for the 'majority'. This being the case, the needs of people from minority groups will always take second place to the white majority. It is not surprising that families sought solutions from within their own communities, and services tended to be developed by the voluntary organizations from within these communities. These organizations were reliant upon funding from a variety of sources and had to compete for resources with other organizations. This funding situation meant that people with learning disabilities from minority ethnic communities tended to receive less funding than their white counterparts. This became particularly evident when the Government made additional money available to close the long-stay hospitals. As a great number of people with learning disabilities from minority ethnic communities did not live in these hospitals, they did not benefit from the funding of community care services as did their white counterparts.

The lack of appropriate services for people with learning disability from minority ethnic communities is therefore well known and the government published a study in 2001 specifically addressing the issue of learning disability and ethnicity (Mir, Nocon & Waqar Ahmed, 2001). Sadly, many problems still exist, although the report does highlight examples of approaches that seek to meet the needs of people with learning disabilities from minority ethnic communities more appropriately.

The main thrust of the report can be summarized in the following points.

- People with a learning disability from a minority ethnic community face discrimination in employment, education, health and social care.

- Negative racial stereotypes and attitudes held by paid carers can contribute to the disadvantage faced by the learning-disabled from minority ethnic communities.
- There is a need to develop further advocacy services and self-advocacy schemes that are flexible and responsive to family structures.
- There are differing views held about concepts such as 'normalization' and 'independence' compared to the white majority and this needs to be acknowledged within service philosophies.
- People with learning disabilities from minority ethnic communities face limited choices in education and employment, which can result in low expectations of services.
- Care staff will need to improve their communication skills to achieve greater cultural competence. This can help people with learning disabilities become more involved in the running of the services they use and the planning of future services.

## Equality and diversity

The issue of institutional racism is a sensitive topic and was rarely acknowledged until the tragic events surrounding the death of Steven Lawrence and the resulting report by Lord McPherson. If care services adopt a 'colour blind' approach to care delivery then some of the care practices within that establishment will be institutionally racist. It is not suggested that the care staff are individually racist, but it is an acknowledgement that a lack of knowledge of religious or cultural beliefs may impact negatively upon the person for whom they are caring.

Throughout this book the notion of partnership has been continually reinforced. It is only through a sensitive, therapeutic care partnership that you will start to appreciate the difficulties that a person with a learning disability from a minority community may have faced or may still be facing in their life. You should understand that most black people in this country experience some disadvantage in aspects of their lives as a direct result of their colour.

You must remember that any care partnership that seeks to place the person with a learning disability at the centre of the care process needs to acknowledge that treating everyone the same does not automatically imply equality and anti-discriminatory practice. This approach is flawed as it does not take into account the special cultural needs of the person with a learning disability. As a paid carer, you will need to appreciate that people from different cultural groups will often be disadvantaged and have their right of self-determination compromised. As a consequence, you will have to plan and deliver comprehensive and sensitive support in order for the person with a learning disability to access mainstream services and help to restore them to optimum health.

In displaying a willingness to acquire new knowledge, skills and attitudes about cultures other than your own, you have an opportunity to enrich your own life, enhance your caring skills and dispel any latent stereotypes and prejudices you may have been unaware you held. By equipping yourself with a deeper understanding of the central components of institutional racism and being sensitive to the issues that oppress people from minority groups, you can begin to plan care in truly equal partnerships that are culturally appropriate for the people in your care.

The following section goes on to discuss some of the cultures you may encounter in your capacity as a carer. It draws heavily upon the work of Karmi (1996) and Henley (1982, 1983).

Ethnic minorities represent a significant part of the population. According to the 1991 Census there are around three million people from minority ethnic communities. The following information is designed to enhance your knowledge about some of the main communities and their cultural beliefs and practices.

## Buddhism

Karmi (1996) offers the explanation of Buddhism as a way of life, incorporating a philosophy and a system of ethics instead of a set of social rules. It revolves around a central tenet, that suffering can be stopped by eliminating selfish desires. Belief in rebirth encourages virtuous behaviour in this life, so that one may make spiritual progress in the next. The ultimate Buddhist goal is to escape the eternal cycle of life and death and reach a higher state of understanding and Nirvana.

Buddhists are expected to observe five precepts.

- Do not kill.
- Do not steal.
- Maintain correct sexual contact.
- Tell the truth.
- Do not use intoxicating substances.

Buddhism emphasizes the importance of love for all living beings and respect for all forms of life, as well as charity, hospitality and self-discipline.

## Religious celebrations

At some time between April and May, at the full moon, Buddhists throughout the world celebrate Wesak, which simultaneously marks the birth, enlightenment, and entry into Parinirvana (complete passing away) of the Buddha. Wesak also marks the Buddhist New Year. Dates are based on a lunar calendar, and are therefore liable to vary. Mahayana Buddhists commemorate the same above events but on three separate days, on 8 April, 8 December and 15 February, respectively. They also celebrate Ullumbana (all souls) and New Year.

## Religious practices

Specific religious practices for Buddhists include meditation and chanting. Incense is often burned during meditation. Some Buddhists fast or abstain from eating meat on the first and fifteenth day of each lunar month, that is when the moon is either full or new. Pilgrimages to the four main sites relating to the life of Buddha, all located in India, are considered of great value.

## Diet

There are no specific dietary regulations, but most Buddhists are vegetarian.

## Death

Cremation is preferred. A Buddhist monk or priest will normally officiate.

## Medical information

Nothing worthy of note.

## Activity

Find out what date Wesak falls upon this year.

## Hinduism

Henley (1983) suggests that Hinduism is the religion practised by 80% of people from India. Hinduism is, however, much more than a religion; it is a social system that gives order to a way of life and is underpinned by a set beliefs, values and religious practices.

Unlike Christianity or Islam, Hinduism has neither a single founder nor a holy book. It is a continually evolving religion shaped by different thoughts and practices. Hindus recognize that there are many different ways in which an individual may worship and that all will reach the same goal.

Hindus believe in the existence of one single supreme spirit, the immortal soul, and the existence of all living things and the cycle of reincarnation. There is a fundamental belief in a cycle of reward and punishment for every thought, with a non-violent code acknowledging the supreme duty of seeking truth.

## Religious festivals

Major Hindu festivals are: Mahashivaratri (the birth of Shiva) in February or March; Ram Navami (birth of Ram and the incarnation of Vishnu) in March or April; Janmastarni (the birth of Krishna) in August or September; and Diwali, the festival of light, in October. Dates will vary slightly according to the cycle of the moon.

## Religion

According to Karmi (1996), Hindu rules will vary according to caste. The higher the caste, the more religious observance is expected. The highest caste, Brahmins, have ultimate responsibility in religious matters. Fasting is usually undertaken by devout Hindus, mainly by women. Some practising Hindus may fast regularly each week, depending on their loyalty to a particular deity or the astrological significance of certain days. Fasting in this sense implies eating only 'pure' foods, such as fruits or yoghurt, rather than complete abstinence.

## Religious practices

Every Hindu has a chosen god and every home will have a prayer room (puja). Worship may take place anywhere, as God is considered omnipresent. However temple worship is customary, and a priest (pujani) may be in attendance to assist in rituals. Pictures and silver or gold idols of gods normally adorn the place of worship, and offerings are often made in the form of food or money. It is therefore important to remember that Hindu people who have a learning disability too may also require a place of worship within their own home. This may prove difficult within a small community home, therefore special arrangements within the home may need to be made to facilitate this practice.

## Diet

The majority of Hindus do not eat meat, meat products (e.g. lard, gravy, etc.) or fish, and many abstain from eating eggs, as these are considered a potential source of life. Milk is always acceptable. Some lower caste Hindus eat meat but not beef, as cows are considered sacred. Pork is not usually eaten as pigs are regarded as unclean. Tea, coffee, garlic and onions are avoided by some Hindus because they are considered excessively stimulating. Alcohol is officially disapproved of but not forbidden.

## Social customs

Spiritual purity and physical cleanliness are extremely important. Modest dress is prescribed for men and women: men must be covered from waist to knees. Hindu women do not like to undress fully for medical examinations, and they also prefer to be examined by female medical staff.

Hindus prefer to wash themselves in running water, so showers are preferable to baths. As in other eastern religions, it is customary for people to remove footwear on entering the home. Smoking is frowned upon but is not forbidden.

## Death

Hindus are normally cremated.

## Medical information

Blood transfusions and organ transplants are permitted.

## Issues of interest

Traditional medicine can be practised alongside conventional medicine.

## Islam

Henley (1982) describes Islam as the religion belonging to Muslims. The literal meaning of the word 'Islam' is submission, therefore a Muslim is a person who submits to the will of God and is at peace with him.

Living a life as a Muslim means following clear-cut rules that cover day-to-day life. This means that although cultures of Muslims in different countries may vary, the basic beliefs and practices of devout Muslims remain the same everywhere. All Muslims' believe the prophet Muhammad to be the final messenger of the one true God. All Muslims' believe that they must observe the five main duties of Islam:

- faith;
- prayer;
- giving alms;
- fasting;
- pilgrimage to Mecca.

Strict Muslims pray five times a day, starting before sunrise and ending at night. During prayer, the head must be facing towards Mecca and the forehead touches the ground. Friday is a religious day and men attend the mosque. A sick person may need privacy during the day at prayer times, assistance in facing Mecca and the washing of face, feet, hand and forearms before prayer. It is not permitted to pray before thorough cleaning with water.

## Diet

Karmi (1996) indicated that Islam permits the consumption of 'halal' meat only. This is meat which has been killed according to Islamic law. Pork products are not eaten and a few sea foods may not be allowed. Alcohol is not allowed in Islam. Water is traditionally taken with meals.

Fasting is required during Ramadan, the ninth lunar month, with no food or drink consumed between sunrise and sunset, although the ill, children, people travelling a long distance where nourishment is necessary for survival and women who are menstruating, are considered exempt. Fasting may also extend to the withdrawal of medications, including injections, during this daylight time.

## Customs

Traditional Muslims may observe Purdah, where the women are clothed from head to foot. In hospital women, may wish to remain as fully clothed as possible and many will choose to be seen only by female health professionals. Men may prefer to remain covered from waist to knee and be cared for only by male staff. Both men and women will generally want water for washing before and after meals as well as for toilet hygiene.

## Gender issues

Attitudes to women vary considerably between the different West Asian countries and between individuals. A few women wear clothing covering the whole body, and are not permitted to work outside the house or drive. Other women may have lifestyles largely indistinguishable from those of the wider community.

## Death

Karmi (1996) suggested that, when dying, a Muslim person may prefer to face Mecca. After death the body is traditionally covered with a sheet. According to Islamic law the body must be buried within 24 hours of death and will need to be ceremoniously washed prior to burial. Many Muslims believe in life after death and that the soul stays near the body until burial. Some families may prefer to take a body home or to the mosque for preparation for burial. A period of public grieving following a burial may vary in duration.

## Medical information

When a person is sick, it is usual for the family to notify all relatives. The sick person is usually happy to receive many visitors.

Transplantation of human organs is permissible under Islam. In some communities, bad news is never told directly to a person for fear of the shock it may cause. The family may be reluctant for a person with a learning disability to learn they are terminally ill. In these cases, you will need to consult with the family.

## Specific health issues

You should consider not using your left hand in touching or giving materials to the Muslim person with a learning disability in your care. The left hand is used for toilet hygiene. Many Muslims do not like their head being touched. This is not a religious but a cultural preference.

## Judaism

Karmi (1996) describes the Jewish community as both a religious and an ethnic group. The Jewish community in Britain is very diverse, reflecting differing degrees of assimilation, religious observance, and geographical origin. There is a strong emphasis on family ties throughout the Jewish community, especially among the orthodox. The community is generally well provided with voluntary organizations that care for elderly and disadvantaged groups such as people with a learning disability.

## Language

English is almost universally spoken in the Jewish community. Yiddish is spoken by some of the elderly and by members of the Orthodox religious community. Hebrew is the language of prayer (and of Israelis). Other languages such as Polish or German are also spoken, depending on the area of origin. Jews from North Africa and parts of the Middle East use Arabic.

## Religious festivals

Among the most important annual events are Rosh Hashanah (New Year), also known as Yom ha-Din (Judgement Day), in September/October and Yom Kippur (the Day of Atonement), which takes place 10 days later. In early spring there is Pesach (Passover), which celebrates the exodus from Egypt, followed by the harvest festival Shavuot (Pentecost) 50 days later. Sukkot (Tabernacles) is the autumn harvest festival. There are several other minor feast days and fasts throughout the year, among them Chanukah or Hanukkah, an eight-day event in mid-December marked by lighting candles, and Purim (the story of Esther). Saturday is the weekly day of rest. These events are based on the lunar calendar, so dates vary from year to year.

## Religious practices

Jewish religious practices are laid down in the Torah (the first five books of the Bible) (Karmi, 1996), and interpreted by the rabbis or religious teachers in the Talmud and other religious texts. Orthodox Jews observe these teachings strictly, while others, such as the progressive reform and liberal groups, make more concessions to modern lifestyles. Many Jews have abandoned ritual practice altogether. Virtually all ritual laws are waived if life is considered to be in danger.

The Sabbath (Shabbat), the Day of Rest, begins at sunset on Friday and ends on Saturday evening. On the Sabbath, Orthodox Jews will not do any type of work, or physical activities, including relatively small tasks, such as carrying a bag, driving, switching a light on or pushing a pram.

Fasting lasts for 25 hours, beginning at sunset on the eve of Yom Kippur. Orthodox patients must be offered alternatives to oral medication, such as injections or suppositories. For them, this day is emotional and highly significant. Some people with a learning disability may also observe other fasts with equal strictness.

# Diet

Dietary regulations are observed to varying degrees by all practicing Jews. Pork and its derivatives and shellfish are strictly prohibited. Other meat is kosher (permitted) provided it has been slaughtered according to Jewish law. Orthodox Jews are not permitted to eat meat and dairy products together or within several hours of each other, and must use separate plates and utensils for them.

According to Karmi (1996), practicing Jews are not supposed to take non-kosher medication unless there are no alternatives; in this case they must be instructed to do so specifically by the doctor and a rabbi. All food has to be specially inspected by a rabbi (except fruit and vegetables), and bears a special label to show that it has been passed.

For the eight days of Pesach (Passover) no leavened bread, cakes or biscuits are eaten. Some medicines may also be forbidden, and special advice from the rabbi will be required by health professionals. During Pesach Orthodox Jews will not eat any food unless specifically supervised.

# Death

Funeral services are relatively simple. Preferably the body should be interred within 24 hours of death. Post mortems are not permitted unless legally required. Following the funeral, close relatives remain at home and refrain from daily activities.

# Medical information

Blood transfusions are permitted. Organ transplants are usually forbidden by Orthodox Jews. However, opinions vary, and decisions may rest with the rabbinic authority.

# Sikhism

The Sikh community (as explained by Karmi, 1996) is both an ethnic and a religious group. Founded by Guru Nanak in the 16th century, the Sikh faith has its roots in Hinduism, but has developed into a separate religion over the course of the following 200 years. Unlike Hindus, Sikhs are monotheistic, worshipping one supreme God, and believe in the equality of all before the creator. However, certain beliefs are shared with Hinduism, notably beliefs in reincarnation and karma.

Religious life revolves around the Sikh temple. Sikhism has always been inextricably bound up with the language, culture and history of the Punjab, in North West India, where 90% of India's Sikhs live and from where most Sikhs in Britain originate.

## Language

The mother tongue of the Sikh community is Punjabi. Most Sikhs have three names: a first name, a religious tide (Singh, meaning lion, for all men and Kaur, meaning 'prince' for all women), and a family name. The family name is not used by devout Sikhs because family names can often imply caste or sub-caste, which Sikhism does not accept. In Britain family names are sometimes used to ease administrative procedures. The accepted form of address is to use the first name followed by Singh for a man, e.g. Mr Arnaffit Singh. Similarly, a woman's first name should always be followed by Kaur, omitting the family surname.

## Religious festivals

According to Karmi (1996) the main Sikh festivals are: Vaisakhi (New Year) on 13 April; Diwali, held in October/November; and Hola, a three-day pageant in February or March The most important commemorative occasions (gurpurbs) are the birthday of the founder of Sikhism, Guru Nanak, and the birthday of Guru Gobind Singh the most revered Sikh warrior and hero. Other important anniversaries include the martyrdom of Guru Arjan and Guru Tegh Bahadur. All these days vary according to the phases of the moon.

For practical reasons, Sunday is the day of collective worship among Sikhs in Britain.

## Cultural issues

Formally baptized Sikh men (Amridharis) wear the five signs of Sikhism, known as the five Ks:

1. kesh (uncut hair);
2. kangha (comb);
3. kara (steel bangle);
4. kirpan (symbolic dagger);
5. kaccha (symbolic undershorts).

A turban (pagri), the most visible badge of Sikh identity, must be worn by all Sikh men, and only small minorities of Sikhs in Britain do not wear one. Long hair is worn in a bun and covered by a rumal or patka (inner turban) in some cases. The kara is an important talisman and is removed with the greatest reluctance. Many devout Sikhs always wear a kaccha, even if only around one leg and some may refuse to undress completely for medical examination. Many Sikhs in Britain have chosen to give up some of the five Ks, but the devout are reluctant to disregard any of them at any time. Sikh women usually cover their hair with a scarf (dupatta) or, in a few cases, with a tight black or white turban.

Traditional dress for men is the pajama and kameez or kurta (long, buttoned shirt with a high collar), and the shalwar kameez for women. In the case of females, they prefer to consult a female doctor, as modesty is important. Generally speaking, Sikhs prefer to wash in running water, in the shower rather than in the bath. Smoking is strictly forbidden.

## Diet

Although Karmi (1996) indicates that meat is not specifically prohibited, many observant Sikhs are vegetarian and do not eat fish or eggs. Meat has to be jhatka or chakar, slaughtered with one stroke. Eating meat according to the halal or kosher method of draining all blood from the animal is strictly prohibited. Some Sikhs, particularly those who have lived with Hindu populations, may avoid eating beef, as cows are respected animals in India. Pork is generally avoided, as it is considered unclean.

## Death

The family is responsible for all ceremonies and rites at death. There are usually no objections to the body being tended by non-Sikhs, but close consultation with the family is essential on all matters of procedure. Sikhs are cremated, if possible within 24 hours of death, and the ashes are scattered in running water.

## Medical information

Post mortems, blood transfusions and organ transplants are permitted.

## African-Caribbeans

Karmi (1996) offers the following exploration of the African-Caribbean culture: 'The term African-Caribbean (or Afro-Caribbean) describes people of African origin who came to Britain from the Caribbean islands, notably Jamaica, Trinidad and Tobago, Grenada, Dominica, Barbados, St Lucia and the British Virgin Islands. There have been people from the Caribbean in Britain since the 17th century, but the majority of migrants were invited to Britain during the 1950s and early 1960s in response to a shortage of manual labour. The majority of African-Caribbeans live in urban areas, mainly in London, the West Midlands, Bristol, and in Lancashire. People of Caribbean origin in Britain face economic hardship and social deprivation, in which racism often plays a part.'

## Language

English is universally spoken and written, but many people speak a dialect or patois, which combines elements of English, Western European and African languages.

## Religion

Most African-Caribbeans are mainstream Christians. Within this group there are well-defined groups of Pentecostalists, Seventh Day Adventists, and Jehovah's Witnesses. A smaller number are Baptists, Anglicans, Methodists or Roman Catholics. Increasing proportions, particularly among the young, are Rastafarians, or are influenced by them.

# Cultural issues

Rastafarians wear their hair long, in so-called 'dreadlocks', which are never combed or cut, but instead tidied with olive oil or coconut oil (Karmi, 1996). Ganjo (marijuana) is commonly smoked for religious purposes and on social occasions, especially among the young.

# Diet

Most Seventh Day Adventists avoid pork and pork products. Some do not drink tea or coffee, because they are regarded as excessively stimulating. Many Rastafarians also avoid pork; others are vegetarians and refuse to eat grape products; some refuse to use salt. Some Rastafarians are vegans and many avoid foods containing additives and preservatives.

# Medical information

Jehovah's Witnesses are opposed to blood transfusions. Sickle-cell disease is a cardinal feature in this community and the incidence of hypertension and stroke is raised among African-Caribbeans in Britain, as is that of diabetes.

## Bangladeshis

Like many other ethnic minorities, Bangladeshis migrated to Britain mainly for economic reasons. Karmi (1996) offers the following insight into the culture. About half the Bangladeshi community in Britain is concentrated in the Borough of Tower Hamlets in the East End of London. The remainder are largely settled in the Borough of Camden, and in the North of England.

One of the most important barriers to improving the health of the Bangladeshi community is language. Although members of the community have strong faith in modern medicine and consult doctors frequently, treatment is often followed incorrectly or left incomplete because of a poor understanding of English, unfamiliarity with prescriptions, and the traditional health beliefs of the person with a learning disability. Faith healing is commonly practised for both physical and mental illnesses alongside conventional medicine.

## Language

The three most commonly spoken languages are Sylheti, English and Bengali and some Bangladeshis also speak Urdu. Sylheti is a dialect of Bengali and is not written. Many of the health problems of this community could be alleviated by effective communication between paid carers and those in their care.

## Cultural issues

Karmi (1996) informs us that men and women have different naming systems. Men traditionally have two or three names: a personal and a religious name, and a last name, which may be a male title or an extended family (clan) name, such as Kha or Chowdhuri. The use of the surname is optional. In some cases, a father's personal name may have been adopted as a British-style surname for administrative purposes in Britain, as individual family surnames are not used in Bangladesh.

Women usually have two names: a personal name such as Amina or Nadia followed by a female title such as Bibi, Begum, Khanum, Khatoon or Kausar. The title is meaningless on its own; Miss or Mrs Bibi is not acceptable, nor is Mrs Begum. A few women also use their husband's or father's name as a surname. Passports may be the only reliable documents showing correct name, spelling and date of birth. Even then, the latter is often inaccurate.

The traditional dress of Bangladeshi women is the sari, worn over a waist-length blouse and a long underskirt. The head is usually covered by the sari or a headscarf (burkalhijab). Young women wear shalwar karneez (long shirt over loose trousers) and/or baggy western dress. Older, devout men wear a skullcap, sometimes together with a karneez (a long shirt) and pajama (baggy trousers).

Chewing pan is a very common custom in Bengali society and is practised by men and women. Pan is a mixture of lime betel leaves, betel nuts and other nuts and grains, and is usually eaten after meals. Adults often combine the above mixture with tobacco leaves. The ingredients are often grown at home, so pan is available easily and cheaply. When chewed, the mixture turns a brilliant red colour and this is considered attractive on the lips of young women. However, pan is associated with a number of health risks. The betel nut is the subject of ongoing research; it is addictive and can cause dizziness and perspiration. Chewing tobacco has the added risk of causing cancer of the mouth, throat and stomach.

## Diet

The traditional Bengali diet is healthy, being rich in fish, vegetables and pulses. Problems arise in Britain when dietary customs change, notably to a higher sugar and lower fibre intake. This results in more dental decay, especially in children, and may well contribute to poorer general health.

## Medical information

Karmi (1996) suggests the incidence of tuberculosis is high in this group. This may be linked to infection and re-infection with travel to and from Bangladesh, where the disease is endemic, and to low socio-economic status.

As is the case for other South Asian groups, there is an increased incidence of coronary heart disease and diabetes.

Peptic ulcer is particularly common among Bangladeshi men and current research is directed at investigating the cause, which may be linked to betel nut chewing, and, in the case of men, aggravated by heavy smoking.

Many Bangladeshis suffer from depression and anxiety as a result of poor housing conditions, unemployment, culture shock and racial harassment. Women are more prone to depression because of their social isolation.

## Chinese

## Language

Mandarin is the official language of the People's Republic of China and Taiwan, and is quite widely spoken in Malaysia and Singapore. Cantonese is the language of the Chinese from Hong Kong, Guandong province of the People's Republic of China, Vietnam and many from Malaysia, Singapore and Christmas Island. Hokkein is quite widely used among those from Malaysia and Singapore, while Hakka is commonly used in Malaysia, Indonesia and Brunei. Teo-chieu is spoken by the majority of Chinese from Thailand.

Lack of eye contact, shyness and passivity are cultural norms and are not necessarily a sign of anything being wrong. Many Chinese do not want to talk to an outsider about their problems, especially psychosocial ones. Many consider saying 'No' impolite and they may go to considerable lengths to avoid saying it.

In some cases, a paid carer's assertiveness may be interpreted as aggressiveness or hostility. You may have to communicate with family members and involve them in the care plan.

## Religion

Rather than subscribing to a single faith, many Chinese in Britain tend to be influenced by a variety of religions, principally Taoism, Confucianism and Buddhism. There is also a sizeable minority of Christians (mainly Roman Catholic, Protestant or Baptist), although these too are influenced by Taoist and Confucian beliefs. Most Christians from Hong Kong are Protestant.

## Cultural issues

Cultural values of major importance are hard work, acceptance of what life brings, respect for and harmonious coexistence with nature, setting the family before individual welfare, education, self-control, self-actualization, interdependence, respect for elders, collectivism and loyalty to the family. Lineal ties are important, and traditionally ancestors were honoured and worshipped. Prescribed roles, obligations and duties influence interactions heavily, as does the need to avoid 'loss of face'. Loss of face brings shame to the whole family, including one's ancestors. Open discussion about sexuality is considered taboo.

## Social structure

Chinese society is traditionally patriarchal, so that men, not women, own property, receive inheritance, and enjoy other powers. This is tending to change. The basic social and economic unit is the family, with parents living with their son and daughter-in-law. Although this is a common practice in some Chinese-speaking countries, it is less common in Australia. People of Chinese descent still have a strong cultural identity and celebrate traditional calendar festivals, especially Chinese New Year. Marriage is still largely within the Chinese community, so community members remain relatively ethnically distinct.

The status of women is in transition. In traditional households, women are subordinate and expected to be passive and obedient to men. Even within this traditional household, however, older women may have considerable power in respect of the running and functioning of a household and the conduct of its members. Younger women now tend to have much greater economic and personal freedom in their daily lives.

## Diet

Traditional Chinese meals include a high intake of fruit and vegetables, and rice and noodles are staples. Diets emphasize balance, and are based on the traditional ideas of yin and yang 'hot' and 'cold' foods. Many Chinese are particularly careful about the foods they eat when they are sick, and avoid 'raw' foods such as salads.

## Death

Some families wrap the body in a special white shroud made from coarse material. Generally speaking, however, the deceased is buried in his or her best clothes. Some elderly people keep their own burial gowns in case their younger relatives will not know how to dress them after their death. Post mortems are not prohibited but are considered undesirable and distressing.

## Medical information

Food, illness and medications are classified, according to the perceived effects on the body, as 'hot' or 'cold'. Health is believed to be a balance of positive (yang) and negative (yin) energy in the body. Chi refers to the life force or energy in the body. Illness may be caused by disharmony of body elements, for example, an excess of 'hot' or 'cold' foods. In this context, 'hot' and 'cold' refers to the effect of the food on the body and not its temperature. Illness resulting from excess 'hot' or 'cold' is remedied by restoring the balance of foods in the diet.

Poor feng shui can result from the impact of the natural and manmade environment on the fortune and well-being of inhabitants. Chinese medicine is an established therapeutic tradition which treats the person as a whole using acupuncture, acupressure and Chinese herbs. Dietary therapy, traditional herbal medicine, Western medicine and supernatural healing (through a fortune teller, feng shui man or temple medium) may also be used.

Approximately 20% of ethnic Chinese are thought to be hepatitis B carriers. The incidence of nasopharyngeal, oesophageal and stomach cancer in China is high. There are indications that these cancers also affect the Chinese population in Britain. Heavy smoking is common, particularly among men.

## Conclusion

In conclusion, this chapter has explored issues of race, culture and religion and the importance they play in people's lives. There is a need for all paid carers working with people who have a learning disability to re-appraise their care practices to ensure people's cultural needs are acknowledged within their plan of care.

## Activity

1. You may wish to re-take the test you completed at the beginning of this chapter.
2. Identify what needs to be taken into account in the service where you are working to ensure it provides services that are culturally competent.

## References

Ayer, S. (1997) Cultural diversity: issues of race and ethnicity in learning disability. In: *Dimensions of Learning Disability*, Gates, B. & Bacock, C. (eds). London: Baillièe Tindall.

Baxter, C., Poonia, K., War, L. & Nardishaw, Z. (1990) *Double discrimination. Issues and services for people with learning disabilities from black and ethnic minority communities*. London: Kings Fund Centre.

Henley, A. (1982) *Caring for Muslims and their Families: Religious Aspects of Care*. London: Health Education Council.

Henley, A. (1983) *Caring for Hindus and their Families: Religious Aspects of Care*. London: Health Education Council.

Karmi, G. (1996) *The Ethnic Health Handbook*. Oxford: Blackwell Science.

McMillan, S. (1992) What are the differences in the patterns of disability, knowledge about services, and the experience of using services between Asian adults with learning difficulties and their carers living in the eastern half of the city of Leicester? MSc thesis, University of Keele.

Mir, G., Nocon, A. & Waqar, A. (2001) *Learning Difficulties and Ethnicity*. Report to the Department of Health. London: HMSO.

# Appreciating family experiences of learning disability

**9**

## Acknowledgement

During the Royal College of Nursing Congress at Harrogate in April 2001, it was my privilege to attend an address given at a fringe event by Richard Jackson, MBE, to nurses involved in the care of people who have a learning disability. I felt humbled as Richard recounted his experience of caring for his son, Steven, especially the way his views always seemed of less value than those of the professional 'experts' involved with Steven's care. There are many different partnerships that exist between paid carer and informal carer but such partnerships are meaningless unless the informal carer's voice is heard and treated with equal respect to the voice of the 'expert'.

Both Nicky and I are indebted to RESCARE for giving permission for this, 'Steven's Story' to be reproduced (Jackson, 2000). *Tom Tait*

## Steven's story

Born between the wars, married during the second, my wife Edith helping to produce khaki cloth and I wearing it until the war's end, we looked towards the future like millions of our generation, thankful that we had been spared and hopeful for its blessings.

Living in a small terrace house in Farnworth, Lancashire, I resumed employment in chemical engineering, with my apprenticeship having been disrupted by service in HM Forces. I took up attendance at night school to ultimately gain, after some nine years, Associate Membership of the Institution of Mechanical Engineers. Edith, putting our home together, prepared to raise a family, for shortly after my demobilisation our first child Rita was born in April 1947. Being born prematurely, there were complications which resulted in her being returned to hospital for two months but all turned out well and she was a beautiful child.

It was three years later, on the 29th May 1950, that our only son Steven arrived, born at home, under the auspices of the midwife, as were all our children and was the fashion in those days. All seemed well and with 'one of each', Edith and I were at peace with the world for what was to be a few short weeks before the euphoria was to dissipate.

Steven started to suffer bouts of screaming and banging his head with his small fists. The doctor and nurses could offer no explanation and showed no concern. Eventually the bouts subsided. There was no hint that anything was seriously wrong but Edith had begun to express unease at Steven's lack of progress. 'He'll grow out of it,' 'All children are different', said friends and relatives. But as our concern increased, we desperately hoped and prayed that they were right.

As Steven approached his first birthday, Edith confronted the doctor with her concern and for the first time she was told that our son would be permanently backward. She felt at that moment a coldness of the unknown, a desire to step out of the fog into which she was sinking but with awareness that the child on her knee was to be loved and protected.

I came home from work that day to find Edith heartbroken and Rita, now four, in tears as she too sensed that something was wrong. Going immediately to our doctor's surgery, I questioned him at length, frustrated at what appeared to be a superficial observation with little in-depth examination. He confirmed Steven's backwardness with little advice as to what to do. It was left to Edith to attend, as did all mothers and their babies, the post natal clinic with one heartrending difference—Steven's card which Edith had to take with her was marked MD—Mental Defective.

We refused to accept the permanence of Steven's condition and did the rounds of specialists, second opinions and even a radio faith healer, praying fervently for a release. During those early years, we clutched at all manner of straws hoping to bring to our son the means to cure his handicap and resolve our increasing distress as we desperately tried to cope with the situation, but it was all to no avail.

There was a slowness to crawl and then to walk. Taking him through toilet training and the accomplishment of accepting his food without covering the area around him were, for us, tremendous steps forward and a relief particularly to Edith and Rita, both of whom bore the brunt of his development. Then, as one particular day dawned, so too did the realisation for Edith and I that Steven's malady was a fact, and a permanent one that we must accept and learn to live with. This recognition changed our attitude from negative to positive and though, with no agency to help, the learning was hard, learn we did.

As a family, it was as though we were different too. The nudges, the looks, the whispers, which were increasingly noticed as Steven grew older and his handicap became more apparent; often bringing us silent tears and sometimes anger. We did not, however, allow this to destroy our faith in ourselves or our son, Steven, and in this we treasured the friends whose help was meaningful. Our initial decision to accept and no longer avoid the challenge did allow us to re-align our sights and to take the days as they came. Whilst we planned our activities around Steven, we tried to ensure that the disruption to our own and our other children's lives was kept to an acceptable minimum. After Steven, we had Glenys and Yvonne and at each birth the anxiety of the seemingly endless pregnancy was relieved by a perfect baby girl.

It was when Steven was three that fate struck us another blow. Having enjoyed an afternoon at the local annual fair, Steven, tired, was in my arms, when suddenly he stiffened and went into a convulsion, vomiting and shaking profusely. The doctor was called when we reached home. Steven had suffered his first epileptic fit and subsequently he was to suffer several a week. We were given no help or advice, other than how to prevent him hurting himself. To see our child in such torment caused us extreme anguish, as we felt powerless to help.

In the meantime Steven, exploded into hyperactivity which tired everyone but him. It was only through determination and dedication, particularly by Edith, that Steven gained a few words of speech, and as he grew it fell to Rita to supervise his play when outside. She often returned in tears following the taunts of other children. Consequently, we phased play periods to allow her time out on her own.

Having moved to Winton, Eccles, our next hurdle came as Steven reached school entry age at five, when Edith presented him to the local primary school. Entry was refused and an appointment was immediately made for Steven to be assessed by the education authority's psychologist. This proved a short-lived affair and after a few of the usual mental tests it was announced that Steven would have to be certified 'uneducable' with responsibility for his care and treatment passing to the health authority. We appealed and got a stay of execution until Steven was seven, in the hope that he might improve; the understanding being, however, that in the interim he could not attend school. Edith courageously accepted this in a hopeful attempt to keep open the door for our son. Again, it was to be in vain.

It was from the school psychologist that we first learnt of the National Association of Parents of Backward Children (now MENCAP) and we joined the local branch, gaining encouragement from the meetings we attended. For the first time we did not feel alone. It was because of the pioneering work of the Association that what were later to be termed occupation centres, were established first by parents in church halls and other locations. These were subsequently taken over and run by the health authorities. However, Steven, not having been assessed as 'uneducable' was not allowed to go to such a centre and remained at home.

I would not want to give the impression that it was all doom and gloom. We were, and are, a close family, and the laughs came as did the tears. For us, while the lows could be very low, the highs were very high indeed. We lived at the extremes of emotion but were each strengthened by our experience.

Our holidays soon avoided boarding houses or hotels. On our first family holiday in Morecambe, the landlady generously agreed to look after our children for the first evening, while Edith and I had an hour or so to ourselves. On our return, we found a dishevelled landlady and a heartbroken Steven, so future holidays were taken in holiday cottages or caravans, where we did our own thing. In later years, we would stagger our holidays with Steven going into respite care while the family had a week on our own. Then, the second week would be taken with Steven, when he enjoyed being the centre of our efforts. This arrangement worked well.

At five years of age, Steven's epileptic fits were continuing and it was an exceptional attack which went on for some hours which necessitated a 999 call. This resulted in Steven being rushed to Park Hospital, Davyhulme, Manchester. Dr Eagan, the paediatrician and her team fought long and hard for Steven and saved him. We agreed to Steven staying for a week of observation by Dr Eagan and for the very first time, we received help, advice and treatment for which, to this day, we are ever grateful. Steven was put on phenobarbitone, which, over the years, has gradually reduced the incidence of his fits. In fact now at 45, he has not had one for four or five years. Over the next few years, Dr Eagan helped us so much. Steven's tonsils were removed, clearing up his continual running nose, and when he was seven, she arranged for him to have plastic surgery on his ears, reducing their prominence. 'Standing out like a cab with the doors open' was the general expression at that time. 'This boy has enough to contend with, let's rectify what we can', the doctor said. This was true enough as a well known character in the TV series Noddy was named 'Big Ears', which prompted children to christen Steven likewise.

On his entry into Wythenshawe Hospital for surgery the nurse bathing him said: 'So you're going to see Mr Champion (the surgeon) are you?' Steven replied, remembering his favourite TV programme: 'Champion the wonder horse!' Following the operation, Steven finally emerged from a swathe of bandages to reveal his ears laid back, which greatly improved his appearance. We were delighted and for a long time Steven was pleased to tell people: 'My new ears, my new ears.' No more were they, nor he, to be the butt of cruel innuendoes.

As Steven's seventh birthday came round so did his re-assessment and the local branch of the National Association for Parents of Backward Children kindly offered to pay for this to be done privately in our own home. It was undertaken by a Dr Fish from Booth Hall Hospital who, with great sensitivity at the conclusion of the assessment, confirmed what we feared. Steven should be certified 'uneducable' (and this time we had no option but to accept. A visit to the health authority headquarters in Preston reassured us that certification would open the way for Steven to go to an occupation centre. After several months and much correspondence this was achieved, and Steven, who was collected each morning and returned each afternoon, attended a centre in Stretford.

For Edith it was at last a welcome relief and one she deserved. Soon our family settled into a more normal routine with Rita and Glenys at school and Steven settled into his centre. Yvonne was born in 1957, a year before we moved to Bramhall, Cheshire, the move being a result of the company for which I was now Works Manager, moving to a new factory at Wythenshawe. Steven was eight.

Still maintaining our membership of the National Association of Parents of Backward Children we transferred to the Stockport branch of the Society where I joined the Committee as a founder member in its formative years. My main function was the placing and emptying of collection boxes in pubs and clubs and I represented the Society in the founding of Stockport Hospitals' League of Friends, with my particular interest being directed to the Offerton House Hospital for people with a mental handicap. In fact, the first colour television in that hospital was donated by the League of Friends.

We applied for Steven to be admitted to an occupation centre in the local area and it was arranged that the head of a unit in Macclesfield would visit our home to assess him. The lady duly arrived but sadly Steven had one of his epileptic seizures during her visit. 'I'm afraid we can't cope with that', she commented, and in spite of our protests, he was refused entry.

The load again fell on Edith and for some months she seemed to cope until suddenly she was admitted to hospital for a minor operation. During Edith's two week absence, Steven attended Brockhall Hospital for people with a mental handicap but on her return the strain of coping with Steven was beginning to tell. Rita (12) and Glenys (6) at their new schools and Yvonne (3) at home were missing out as pressures increased.

Coming home from the office each day it was literally to pick up the pieces as Edith headed for a breakdown and our girls cried over smashed toys. Our family was disintegrating, as Steven erratically ran here and there unable to concentrate for long and with all our attempts to occupy him having no effect. Steven was taken over by continuous bouts of hyperactivity and Edith was no longer able to cope. He slept little and we had to remove anything that might constitute a danger. Our lives were in total and unending upheaval.

It was at this point that Edith and I realised that the time had sadly come to put the lives of our girls first, and the decision was made that some form of residential care had to be sought. On our journey to our GP, Steven wet himself twice, such had his control deteriorated. On entering the surgery, the doctor asked me to let Steven go, I did and in a few seconds his office looked like a bomb had hit it, as the telephone went one way, his files another. Together we restrained Steven and looking at me the doctor asked, 'What do you want me to do?'. 'We can't go on doctor', I replied, 'Our family is suffering more than is reasonable. My wife and I feel he needs residential care with trained staff able to cope with him.' 'I think you are right', the doctor commented, 'but you had to say it with no prompting from me. I will make arrangements for him to go into a special hospital as soon as a place is available.'

While awaiting his move into residential care, it was discovered that Steven had a diseased kidney. This had come to light as a result of

Steven's participation in a national research programme agreed some years earlier with Dr Eagan at Park Hospital, Macclesfield. Although we were aware that involvement in this research was unlikely to benefit Steven, we felt it right to help as the results of the research might benefit others, particularly future generations.

Our hearts dropped when we were informed of Steven's diseased kidney. He was kept in hospital over Christmas and when we visited him on Christmas Day, the specialist asked to see us and we received the news that thankfully the kidney was not diseased but had a blockage which could be removed with no ill effects. Our relief moved us to tears. We then joined the Christmas revels at the kind of party that only a hospital can put on and where, as is the custom, the specialist carved the turkey.

Steven then went into the Royal Manchester Children's Hospital for the operation which was successful. After the operation, his arms were put in splints and tied to stop him pulling at the tubes. He was particularly proud of the bottle beneath his bed and he made sure that all the visitors had a good look at it. Edith and I would sit at his bedside until late into the night coaxing him to sleep to relieve the staff.

When we eventually got the call to bring him home, it was more a call for help from staff at a loss as to how to cope with Steven. Visitors bringing fruit, sweets, etc., to the ward were shared amongst the patients. As I opened the door to the ward, the sight that met my eyes is with me still. Steven was sitting surrounded by fruit of all kinds and tucking in—a bite here and a nibble there. On seeing me with his bag of clothes, he let out a cry of joy, tore to his locker and proceeded to empty it. Dressed and ready to go he took my hand. As I was thanking the nurses, quite suddenly and unexpectedly, Steven went to each nurse and raised his face for a kiss. A few handkerchiefs popped out to remove the odd tear. Steven turned for home with an apple and orange stuffed into his pockets.

With Steven now aged ten, a vacancy arose at Swinton Hospital for children with a mental handicap, and with heavy heart we had to let Steven go. It was the most traumatic moment of our lives and was an experience I would wish on anyone.

With one hundred and sixty children, equally divided between boys and girls, they lived in what was an old reform school, one wing for boys and another for girls. Ages ranged from babies to sixteen, with some older and waiting until vacancies for adults arose elsewhere. Mr Williams, the Superintendent, and his wife the Matron, had living quarters in the hospital, which was situated in the centre of Swinton adjacent to Swinton's Town Hall and the nearby Parish Church. A school was located within the hospital grounds.

The format of our lives changed completely. The working days, nights and weekends were now within a more relaxed family atmosphere without the frenzy of living, into which the past years had gradually and subconsciously plunged us. We were determined that Steven's welfare was not to be the price—and we established the pattern that was to take us through the years. I collected Steven every Friday evening, returning him on Sunday, and he came home for all the usual holidays.

Refreshed by the respite during the week, we were to give him our undivided attention when he was home. Our three daughters grew up within this life style and they too benefited. Edith and I concluded that they should be kept free of any decisions regarding Steven. They were entitled to live their own lives uninhibited by any feeling of responsibility, with each of them free to involve themselves to their own inclination. There was never any pressure brought to bear but Edith and I have been proud of the way they have responded to their brother's needs for love and understanding. There is no doubt that he will always have a part in their lives.

Within a matter of weeks, Edith and I approached Mr Williams with a view to starting at the hospital a Parents and Relatives Group that could raise funds to enhance the lives of the children in their care. Mr Williams agreed and following a letter to all the families involved, we were able to establish a Welfare Society with myself as its Honorary Chairman, and a small committee. Funds were raised by all manner of means, not least our Annual Garden Fete attended over the years by celebrities from the entertainment world: Daphine Oxenford (Coronation Street), Wendy Williams and Hugh David (Knight Errant), the Royal Brothers, who were wrestlers, and many others. Christmas parties, birthday gifts, outings, circus and pantomime visits were all part of the way Swinton Hospital was opened up to the community, and the public responded by giving us the financial means to do our work. After five years as Chairman and then another five as President, it was time to take our leave as Steven was transferred to Cranage Hall Hospital, Cheshire at the age of nineteen. We had made many friends, including the residents, and whenever our paths crossed in future years, the memories would flood back of the pleasures brought to their childhood days.

Steven settled down well in Cranage with its school, recreational, social and other services and we were well satisfied with the quality of life it provided for its four hundred or so residents. We continued, of course, to bring Steven home at weekends and for holidays.

It was in 1981, when Steven was thirty one, that we became alarmed. When home at the weekend, Steven would suddenly burst into tears for no apparent reason, Enquiries revealed nothing until we pressed the matter and discovered that Steven and about seven other residents were being segregated for meals and attending 'special' training sessions. They were stopped from going to the workshop or school. After a confrontation with the management, we were informed that our sons and daughters were being prepared to live independently in the community. We had never been consulted or even informed but after prolonged consultations, with myself as spokesman for the parents involved, we drew up and agreed with the authority a document relating to parental rights in the decision making process.

I eventually became Honorary Chairman of the Cranage Hall Parents, Relatives and Residents Welfare Society in 1982 but as the hospital had an excellent League of Friends, we reconstituted the Society with the specific aim to serve and protect the interests of its residents and their families, in view of the new policy of community care and hospital closures now looming on the horizon.

However, it was becoming clear that moves were afoot which sought to sidestep or ignore our views and opinions as parents or relatives; consequently our Society grew rapidly in numbers as others joined because of their growing concern. As a member of MENCAP, I sent a letter to the Executive Committee in London, seeking information as to the rights of families whose dependent relative was cared for in hospital. This drew a disappointing and unhelpful response, merely suggesting that we should seek publicity.

It was then that I recognised the fact that, within the hospital care system for people with a mental handicap, at that time some 40,000 people, the opinion of thousands of families was not being represented. Consequently, I came to the conclusion that this needed a National Society to provide a platform for their voice to be heard, and to enable parents and relatives to play a credible role in the decision making process.

It was in June 1984 that I was able to take early retirement at the age of sixty one, having served my company as Works Manager and Engineer for some thirty-three years. My retirement proved fortuitous in the light of events, for they was to change yet again the shape of the lives of Edith, our family and myself. It was, for me, the beginning of an entirely new, unpaid, excitingly challenging 'career' but one of great satisfaction.

I started to contact other groups in similar hospitals whenever I could wrest the information from authorities. Members of these groups expressed similar concerns to our own. During my various comings and goings I had heard of a residential village community called 'Ravenswood' in Berkshire, the Principal of which was Professor Stanley Segal, OBE. Edith and I visited Ravenswood, were impressed by what we saw, and Professor Segal kindly agreed to come to Cranage and speak to members of our Cranage Parents and Relatives group about the Ravenswood community. His response to this invitation was: 'When parents call, who am I to refuse?'. I remember picking Professor Segal up at Crewe Station and having a hurried chicken salad lunch propped on our knees in a packed Knutsford Service Station before proceeding to Cranage. It was then that I outlined to Professor Segal my ideas for a village community at Cranage. I envisaged it as we had seen Ravenswood. This could be done by retaining Cranage's support services but replacing the existing villas with purpose-built bungalow living units.

The subsequent meeting went well and our members, the parents and relatives of Cranage's residents, were unanimous in their acceptance of the village community concept. One week later, I received a letter from Professor Segal in which he said that if I did decide to form a National Society of the kind I had described, then he would like to be included in any initiative I took to this end. That was all the encouragement I needed. On the 14th November 1984, I persuaded the Committee of the Cranage Hall Parents, Relatives and Residents Welfare Society, at a meeting in my home, to become a Steering Committee for a National Society. The name I had chosen and which was agreed was National Society for Mentally Handicapped People in Residential Care (RESCARE for short). The idea for the name came at 3.00 a.m. one morning, much to the consternation of Edith! I became its founding Honorary Chairman and the committee comprised Mr R Cannon, Mrs M Hopwood and Mr D Fudge, with Professor Segal appointed as our President.

For twelve months we contacted other groups, spoke at meetings and then with 25 parents' relatives groups in various hospitals having affiliated to us, we held an inaugural meeting in Stockport Town Hall on the 28th September 1985. The Society, its name and its constitution were ratified; Professor Segal was elected Honorary President; I was elected Honorary Chairman with three Vice Chairmen, and an Executive Committee was established. RESCARE was in business!

RESCARE became a registered charity in June 1986, our objectives being, to promote the relief and welfare of people with a mental handicap in all types of residential care establishments, and to secure a wide range of residential care options, including residential and village communities; the latter evolving within suitable hospitals.

The growth of RESCARE was phenomenal. Through its quarterly newsletter (RESNEWS), it presented its case. Our early years of welfare work at campaigning were funded entirely through the fees, subscriptions and donations from affiliated groups, family and individual members. Over the years, we have had five lobby meetings at the Houses of Parliament, with a Minister speaking on four occasions. We filled the Grand Committee Room at Westminster to overflowing when parents and relatives were at last given a opportunity to put their voice on a national platform.

In January 1989, we were able to move the Society's headquarters from our family home, where we had become increasingly submerged by campaigning paraphernalia, typewriter, copying machine, etc., to our present office in Stockport. We were able to engage two part-time employees and life at home became somewhat more ordered for Edith and me.

In the meantime, the campaign to have Cranage Hall Hospital evolve into a village-type community grew, with quarterly Spotlight newsletters informing and presenting the wishes of its members. The campaign was supported vigorously by MPs, Ann and Nicholas Winterton and Gwyneth Dunwoody, by local authorities and local MENCAP societies. By holding meetings, consultations and more meetings, we endeavoured to counter the manoeuvrings of a bureaucratic system and its endless replacement of officials whose main objective was to close the hospital.

We succeeded in persuading Stephen Dorrell MP, when Parliamentary Under-Secretary of State for Health, to visit the hospital. It was no accident that several of the facilities he had hoped to see, including the school and swimming pool, were locked and the keys unavailable. He intimated that he would draw his own conclusions.

Like many parents, we continued to place Steven's name on the waiting lists of voluntary organisations running residential or village communities, for we were increasingly concerned as to Steven's future when we were no longer alive and able to monitor it. It seemed that authorities and their officials were simply unable to grasp the values that tied caring parents to their dependent son or daughter. Much to our relief in March 1990, Steven was offered a place at the Brookvale Community in Prestwich near Manchester. It delivers to Steven, and another seventy residents, a fullness and quality of life which is second to none and which would be difficult to achieve elsewhere. It offers Steven the opportunity for individual achievement and satisfaction, coupled with the privacy afforded by having his own large bedroom with en-suite facilities, built-in furnishings and personal belongings around him. For our Steven, it has opened many doors which are appropriate to his abilities. For Edith and I it brings a peace of mind. We participate fully in his life in an environment that has given our son what we had always longed for—the security of a future that will serve him and his family of friends at Brookvale well. He, and we, have been given back our future; his, God willing, well beyond ours and for that we are thankful.

I had served as Honorary Chairman of the Cranage Hall Parents, Relatives and Residents Welfare Society since 1982, heading the campaign for its evolution into a village community. With Steven now in Brookvale and with my increasing commitment to RESCARE, it was felt by Edith and I that now was the time to ease the pressures by handing over the reins at Cranage to another and concentrating my efforts on RESCARE and any influence it could achieve. This I did at the end of 1990.

RESCARE continued to prosper and its parliamentary lobby meeting in November 1990 addressed by Minister Stephen Dorrell played a major part in the government spelling out in June 1991, the wide range of residential care options acceptable to government, including residential and village communities.

RESCARE delegates, including Patrons Baroness Cox, Lord Pearson, Lord Renton and RESCARE officers, including myself, met a succession of Ministers and Department of Health officials.

This pressure also played no small part in the then Secretary of State, Virginia Bottomley, subsequently giving direction and guidance on the matter of Right of Choice. This directive drew attention to the importance of allowing a choice as to which kind of residential care was suitable to the user, and where he/she was unable to make such a choice, that the decision should be passed to the carer, including parents or relatives.

It was gratifying when RESCARE received a request for affiliation from the national parents/relatives organisations in New Zealand and Australia and it was in 1993 that the organisation in New Zealand took the title RESCARE New Zealand. In the New Year's Honours List, which was announced on 31 December 1993, I was privileged and delighted to be appointed a Member of the Order of the British Empire for services to people with a mental handicap. I was, of course, especially pleased for Edith and our family, without whose support I could have done little. Most important was the honour and recognition it brought to RESCARE and everyone involved in and supportive of its work.

I was fortunate to receive the MBE on their behalf from the Queen on the 16th March 1994, with Edith and our grandchildren Paul and Claire on the front row of the guests; Rita, Glenys and Yvonne foregoing that honour but spending the two days with us in London. It was a moment in our lives shared by our family and by so many from all walks of life who took time out to send their congratulations and best wishes—some we didn't even know. It was a moment that so many other families deserve.

In September 1994 Edith and I, at the invitation of RESCARE New Zealand and CIPAID Australia, embarked on an extensive four week speaking tour of those countries, climaxing at the Annual General Meeting of each organisation.

Our itinerary took us to venues in Auckland, Wellington, Dunedin, Nelson, Christchurch then Melbourne. It was a busy but satisfying experience. In both countries we met government ministers, the media and many families such as our own before spending an extra week resting in the Glass Mountains of Queensland with old friends who also had a boy with Down's Syndrome.

Back in the UK, an important event took place in April 1995. Seeds were perhaps sown then that could contribute to the pendulum swinging back from its extreme ideological to a more practical and more commonsensical position with respect to the care of people with a mental handicap. It was thanks to the untiring efforts of our Patron Baroness Cox, aided by Lord Pearson of Rannoch (RESCARE President), who produced a booklet 'Made to Care—The case for residential and village communities for people with a mental handicap'.

With a foreword by our Patron Lord Renton, it is an exposition of great value. It was launched in Westminster's Jubilee Room on the 3rd April 1995.

'Made to Care' is an important contribution to the debate and one that had an effect. John Bowis, Minister at the Department of Health, announced that an evaluation was to be conducted into the different types of residential provision, including the village community concept. It is a welcome initiative that we trust will be speedily accomplished if hospital sites and their potential value as village communities are not to be lost for ever. We have again asked for a moratorium on hospital closures and/or the sale of their sites pending an evaluation of the research. So the campaign goes on, with RESCARE standing firm behind family wishes. Our membership now reflects equally, those whose dependent relative is within a hospital care system, and those who are cared for in the family home or community-based facilities.

It is a campaign which, for Edith and I, has been fought from the day, now so distant, that was to affect our lives—the 29th May 1950. Along the way we have made so many, many friends. It is the story of thousands of families such as our own across the world who are seeking a secure future for their sons and daughters whose vulnerability is unquestioned, whose need for care and support is life-long and whose quality of life is dependent on others.

As Professor Segal, our late President, said of Ravenswood when he was its Principal: 'It is an island of sanity surrounded by a sea of madness.' Edith and I fully appreciate also the help and understanding of many friends, who have not suffered such a handicap within their own family but who are so willing to contribute in a variety of ways to serve the best interests of all people so disabled and dependent.

We, of the generation born between the wars, who have a son or daughter who has a mental handicap, are often accused of being over-protective, overconcerned with long-term security of care and preoccupied with the taking of risks. The reality is that having been a generation which struggled to establish a comprehensive range of residential options and support services (i.e. group homes, hostels, residential and village communities, respite and day centres, day and residential special schools), we are now fighting the danger of them being swept away on a wave of ideological rhetoric and politically correct dogma.

Steven's future is secure and it is our wish, God willing, to continue the struggle to attain a similar peace of mind for the many families not as fortunate as our own. This then has been our story which we hope will provide encouragement, reassurance and help to other families with a son, daughter or relative with a mental handicap.

## Reference

Jackson, R. (2000) *Bound to Care: An Anthology: family experiences of mental handicap*, Jackson, R. (ed.). Dundee: In House Publications.

# Valuing people: partnerships in care

| |
|---|
| Introduction |
| Children with a learning disability and their families |
| The new vision |
| Offering more choice and control |
| Supporting informal carers |
| Better health for people with learning disabilities |
| Housing |
| Fulfilment |
| Partnerships |

## Introduction

In March 2001 the Government published a white paper to shape the future of care to people with learning disabilities: 'Valuing People—A New Strategy for Learning Disability for the 21st Century' (Department of Health, 2001).

The white paper makes a number of recommendations for the future of learning disabilities in England. Devolution has meant that Scotland, Wales and Northern Ireland will be bringing forward their own recommendations. At the time of writing, these recommendations have not been published. This chapter therefore seeks to explore how the general themes contained within the White paper can shape future services for people with a learning disability, no matter where they live. The discussions will need to be viewed in context with any geographical/demographical issues subsequent reports may highlight.

The changes 'Valuing People' seeks to make may also require you to change your practice to ensure you provide the appropriate opportunities for people in your care to live fulfilling and independent lives as part of a local community.

Following completion of this chapter you will be able to:

- appreciate the problems and challenges surrounding the delivery of care services to people with a learning disability;
- understand how new service structures will shape future provision.

The government suggests that current services for people with learning disabilities within the UK are not consistent and are deficient in some areas which include:

- poorly coordinated services for families with a child who has a learning disability;
- poor planning for children moving from children to adult services;
- not enough support for informal carers, especially those caring for children with complex needs;
- people with learning disabilities having little say in many aspects of their lives;
- people with learning disabilities having unmet health care needs;
- little choice in housing options for people with learning disabilities;
- poor day services, which do not reflect individual requirements;
- limited employment opportunities;
- the needs of people with learning disabilities from minority ethnic communities are often overlooked;
- services differ throughout the country;
- often the statutory bodies who deliver care to people with learning disabilities do not work in real partnership with informal carers or people with learning disabilities.

There are four key principles that underpin the proposals contained within the White paper:

1. rights;
2. choice;
3. independence;
4. inclusion.

Each deficiency will now be discussed and summarized in line with the main recommendations.

## Children with a learning disability and their families

Children with learning disabilities can face many barriers to social inclusion. Research studies (Tait, Beattie & Dejnega, 2002) have demonstrated that services to children with complex needs can be poorly coordinated and lead to carers feeling frustrated with the way services are delivered to their children.

Initiatives such as 'Service Co-ordination' can give carers greater opportunities to have more control over what services their children receive and how these are delivered. Informal carers and professionals can work together in more equal partnerships. Such partnerships can be mutually valued and beneficial. Informal carers can become much more active in organizing their child's care and this leads to greater motivation in informal caring as well as greater job satisfaction for professional carers.

'Valuing People' recognizes that the same health services you may call upon from time to time should be available to children with learning disabilities. As a result of the complex needs that children with a learning disability may have, the number of professionals involved with their care may be many. A robust system of coordination needs to be in place to ensure that everyone knows what each of them is doing to support the family. It is therefore essential that professionals work in such partnership with informal carers to ensure children gain maximum support to enhance their quality of life, while living with their families or in other appropriate settings.

There are a number of existing government initiatives to support children, including 'Meeting Special Educational Needs: A Programme for Action' (Department for Education and Employment, 1998) and the 'Connexions' service (Department for Education and Employment, 2000). The White paper seeks to make children with a learning disability a priority group so that they are supported when they move into adult life.

A separate report relating to families who have a learning-disabled member living at home has been published as part of the government's review (Ward, 2001).

## The New Vision

Two further pieces of legislation underpin the government's drive to change the shape of service provision. The four main principles of Rights, Choice, Independence and Inclusion are supported by the Human Rights Act (1998) and the Disability Discrimination Act (1995). The acts apply equally to all people with learning disabilities.

New funds are to be made available that will be targeted upon specific initiatives which include:

- the modernization of day services;
- facilitating people with a learning disability to move from long-stay hospitals to more appropriate community-based accommodation;
- developing supported living approaches for people living with older, informal carers;
- developing specialist local services for people with learning disabilities who have challenging behaviour;
- the development of integrated facilities for children with severe disabilities and complex needs.

## Offering more choice and control

Some of the discussions contained in this book have served to highlight how little control people with a learning disability have over their lives. This was also true for Steven's parents (see Chapter 9), who felt powerless in their dealings with some professionals.

The government's aim is to give people with learning disabilities as much control as possible over their lives and the services that support them. Two strategies will be employed to facilitate this.

### Direct payments

This is a new way of providing support to people with a learning disability. Rather than the care agency receiving funding from the relevant authority to provide care services to a person with a learning disability, the person themselves will receive payment directly. They will then, in turn, purchase the service that they want. This will give the person with a learning disability greater control over their life.

For people with a mild learning disability this initiative will empower them to take greater responsibility for their care and enhance existing relationships with their paid carers, as they will be working in much more equal partnerships when planning support services. People with a learning disability who have a profound learning disability and/or complex needs will require a great deal of support to access and benefit from this system.

## Person-centred planning

You will already be familiar with this concept from the discussions in Chapter 4. As people with a learning disability take their rightful place within society, they may receive support in varying degrees from a number of voluntary and statutory organizations. If they are to achieve maximum benefit from everyone who is involved in their care, it is essential that a mechanism is in place to coordinate the efforts of all. Such a person-centred approach can help deliver real change to the life of the person with a learning disability, as it provides a single, multi-agency framework for achieving this.

## Supporting informal carers

Caring for a person who has a learning disability is a lifelong commitment. You should remember that there will be many positive aspects of caring, but there are also disadvantages for families who are caring for a member who has a learning disability. Beresford (1995) identified the following:

- high levels of stress;
- lack of finances;
- poor health;
- feelings of isolation;
- problems with housing;
- breakdown in relationships.

A package of financial support is being made available by the government to help with some of these problems, but money alone will be insufficient. A national learning disability information centre and helpline will be opened to give informal carers access to help and support. Proactive strategies will be implemented that identify older informal carers and those from minority ethnic communities, to ensure specific help and support are targeted to families.

## Better health for people with learning disabilities

The respective chapters that focused upon health (Chapters 6 and 7) have demonstrated that people with learning disabilities will have greater health needs than the rest of the population. They have the same right of access to mainstream health services as other people. A new role for paid carers, called Health Facilitator, is being developed to help ensure that people with learning disabilities receive the health care they need. Health Facilitators will work as an integral member of the community learning disability team.

The facilitation of improved health will require each person with a learning disability to be registered with a GP and to have their own Health Action Plan.

## Housing

People with learning disabilities and their families tend to have fewer options about where they live compared to the general population. The government has set a target of the year 2004 for the closure of all long-stay hospitals. Local housing associations will be encouraged to create more flexible housing opportunities.

## Fulfilment

Day-care services for adults have been criticized, as their size and routines can often mean that they cannot cater for every individual need a person with a learning disability may have. It is important that people with learning disabilities are helped to lead full and purposeful lives in their communities and develop a range of different living skills, including leisure interests, friendships and relationships. Day services will therefore need to re-configure the services they provide to ensure that opportunities are created for people with learning disabilities to develop competence in these area.

This too will be the case for educational and employment opportunities. Greater access will be created to adult education through the Learning and Skills Council and the government will set new targets for increasing numbers of people with learning disabilities in paid employment.

## Partnerships

Throughout this book the central theme has been the development of meaningful partnerships between informal carer, paid carer and the person who has a learning disability. Effective partnership working by all agencies is the key to achieving social inclusion for people who have a learning disability.

The government has identified the promotion of stronger, local partnerships as a pivotal initiative in achieving true social integration. These new structures will be called Partnership Boards and consist of a number of key agencies who have a responsibility for providing services to people with learning disabilities at a local level. At a national level a learning disability task force will have the responsibility to take forward key recommendations of 'Valuing People'. The task force will monitor and support the implementation of the recommendations throughout England.

## Conclusion

In summary, the vision contained in this chapter for people with learning disabilities is based upon the principles of rights, choice, independence and inclusion. These principles should underpin and drive any service for people with a learning disability.

To achieve meaningful integration of people with a learning disability into our society will require changes to existing relationships. At the 'micro' level paid carers, informal carers and the person with a learning disability will need to develop more equal, mutually respectful relationships where power is shared and greater trust developed. This will provide a true care partnership in which the person with a learning disability remains at the centre of a therapeutic process, which offers greater control of their life.

At the 'macro' level the agencies involved in commissioning and providing services to people with learning disabilities can work within structures that facilitate integrated strategies within more effective formal partnerships. This will require these agencies to work in new ways with each other and create new and better services for people with learning disabilities, who are one of the most socially excluded groups within the United Kingdom.

## References

Beresford, B. (1995) *Expert Opinions: A national survey of parents caring for a severely disabled child*. York: The Policy Press.

Department for Education and Employment (1998) *Meeting Special Educational Needs: A Programme for Action*. London: HMSO.

Department for Education and Employment (2000) *Connexions: the Best Start in Life for Every Young Person*. London: HMSO.

Department of Health (2001) *Valuing People—A New Strategy for Learning Disability for the 21st Century*. cm5086. London: HMSO.

Tait, T., Beattie, A. & Dejnega, S. (2002) Service Co-ordination: a successful model for the delivery of multi-professional services to children with complex needs. *Nursing Times Research* **7(1)**: 19–32.

Ward, C. (2001) *Family Matters: Counting Families In*. London: HMSO.

# Index

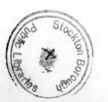